# SCENTUAL TOUCH

# SCENTUAL TOUCH

# TOUCH

## A Personal Guide to Aromatherapy

### JUDITH JACKSON

#### Illustrated by Richard Ely

HENRY HOLT AND COMPANY     New York

Text copyright © 1986 by Judith Jackson.
Illustrations copyright © 1986 by Richard Ely.
All rights reserved, including the right to reproduce
this book or portions thereof in any form.
Published by Henry Holt and Company, Inc.,
521 Fifth Avenue, New York, New York 10175.
Published simultaneously in Canada.

Library of Congress Cataloging in Publication Data
Jackson, Judith.
Scentual touch.
Bibliography: p.
Includes index.
1. Massage.   2. Essences and essential oils—
Therapeutic use.   I. Ely, Richard.   II. Title.
RM721.J32   1986        615.8'22        85-27164
ISBN 0-03-006763-4

First Edition
Designed by Susan Hood
Printed in the United States of America
10 9 8 7 6 5 4 3 2 1

ISBN 0-03-006763-4

*This book is dedicated to all those seeking to add a new
dimension of well-being and pleasure to their lives,
and to my husband and sons whose love and
support have meant so much to the
creation of this book.*

One touch of nature makes the whole world kin.

—William Shakespeare
*Troilus and Cressida*

# CONTENTS

# ACKNOWLEDGMENTS

Thank you seems such a small word for the friendship, talent, and creative energies of: Vicki Lindner, who deserves a lifetime of free Aromatherapy treatment for her editorial assistance; Richard Ely, artist extraordinaire; and Tina Grant, art director.

*I am also deeply grateful to the following advisers whose professional assistance has been invaluable: Dr. William Cain, John B. Pierce Foundation Laboratory, Yale University; Monell Chemical Senses Center, University of Pennsylvania; Edwin T. Morris, instructor in the Cosmetics, Fragrances, Toiletries Department of the Fashion Institute of Technology and consultant to the New York Botanical Gardens; Meredith O'Hara, massage therapist; Roure Bertrand DuPont, producer of natural essential oils, Grasse, France, and Teaneck, New Jersey; Madame Micheline Arcier, Aromatherapist, London, England; Alma Louise Lowe, Ph.D., my aunt and a distinguished woman of letters.*

# SCENTUAL TOUCH

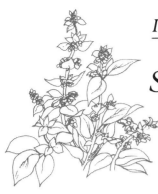

## INTRODUCTION

# SCENTUAL DISCOVERY

In 2,000 B.C., Babylonian kings reveled in Aromatherapy's sensual delights. I discovered the beneficial effects of massage with scented oils for the first time one rainy London afternoon fifteen years ago.

I had arrived in London exhausted from a hectic European business trip. A close friend, who knew of my longtime addiction to massage, suggested I unravel my cat's cradle of jangled nerves with an Aromatherapy treatment at the famous Micheline Arcier salon. I hadn't heard of Aromatherapy and was surprised that any type of massage had escaped my notice.

My friend explained that Madame Arcier had been the protégé of a famous Parisian doctor, Jean Valnet, who had rediscovered the age-old healing properties of essential oils while treating injured soldiers during World War I. She had transplanted Aromatherapy from Paris to London during the 1950s. Aromatherapy was not only an extremely pleasurable form of massage, but a unique method of health and beauty treatments using essential oils and herbs. Gradually, this new French massage system became a discreet London sensation, and a wide range of knowledgeable health enthusiasts, from the titled to the gainfully employed, made up Salon Arcier's privileged clientele. My friend had visited the renowned Madame Arcier, hoping that Aromatherapy treatments would restore her blemished skin. Not only had she seen near-miraculous results, but she found that her entire state of health had improved as well. She had become one of the salon's most confirmed devotées.

Worn out from my travels, I was ready to experience Aromatherapy for myself. I arrived at the lavendar facade of the salon, full of anticipation. A whiff of the aromatic atmosphere, a glance at the shelves of mysterious-looking little brown bottles that held the rare and perishable essential oils, and I found myself thoroughly intrigued. Madame Arcier entered the treatment room with a cheery "Bonjour!" She seemed to embody the healing art she practiced—her skin was firm and fresh-looking, making her seem younger than her years; her blue eyes were startlingly clear and perceptive as if they had already deciphered my thoughts and problems. The Gallic charm of this tall and commanding woman immediately dispelled some of the clouds from the foggy London atmosphere, and my overburdened mind.

She asked me to lie down on a well-padded couch, and covered me with layers of pink towels and blankets, which were then neatly folded back to reveal my bare body. From the moment Madame Arcier placed her strong, warm hand on my tense back, I knew that I had found a new addiction.

As the powerful treatment got under way, it relaxed and calmed my badly frayed nerves and released my tight muscles. I could almost feel the scented oils she was using seeping into my skin, making it feel nourished and supple. The clean fragrance of pure lavender, the faintly exotic sandalwood, the rosy geranium, all titillated my sense of smell, summoning up visions of mythical gardens and forests primeval. Strangely, these subtle perfumes seemed to augment the effectiveness of the massage; they seemed to alter the way my body *felt*, giving me a revitalized, sensual awareness. Tingles and warm surges appeared in areas of my body quite distant from the place where Madame Arcier's skillful hands were actually working. Pressure on my toes was causing my nose to run. When my stomach gurgled in response to mid-back massage, Madame advised, "You must chew more! Remember, you have no teeth in your digestive tract!" She was able to assess my body's overall condition by reading the skin, muscle, and nerve responses to her touch.

During the treatment Madame Arcier asked some pointed questions about the pace of my life, my diet, and my sleeping patterns. Under the releasing sweep of her persuasive hand, I found myself confiding much about the pressures of my position as vice-president of marketing and communications for a large corporation—the demanding job that had brought me to London. I also told her about my interest in preventive health and nutrition, about my night courses in biology, and about the many books I'd read on these subjects. Between groans, as Madame found and untied a knotted fiber in my tension-stiffened neck, I described the problems of being a divorced, single mother in New York City, and spoke of my concern about raising my two little boys while I was working so hard.

By the time Madame completed the treatment by placing her hands flat on the soles of my feet, I felt as if an invigorating electrical charge were surging into my body, yet, at the same time, I was totally relaxed. Was Madame Arcier a good witch, performing miracles with her personal touch? Or was the art she practiced—Aromatherapy—the answer to the needs of all of us who find it so difficult to climb off a whirling merry-go-round of never-ending pressures and obligations? In the years that have passed since the first treatment, I have discovered that the answer to both questions is *yes*.

When I finally managed to rouse myself from my nirvana-like calm, I walked, almost floating, into Madame's consulting room, where she gave me a list of suggestions for bathing in oil-scented water, self-massage, diet, herbal teas, and specific mixtures of essential oils that would help boost and improve my health and energy level. As I reluctantly left her fragrant oasis of calm and caring, carrying small shopping bags of face, body, and bath oils and herbal teas, I was determined to pursue the Aromatherapy way to looking and feeling better. After that, whenever I was in London, I returned to Salon Arcier for Aromatherapy treatments. Eventually I decided to master the art of Aromatherapy, so I could practice it myself. An editorial assignment was all the encouragement I needed.

Several years ago, the health editor of *Harper's Bazaar* asked me to write an article about Aromatherapy, at that time virtually unknown to the American public. Naturally, my first research task was to call Micheline Arcier. During our conversation, Madame mentioned that she was now offering professional training courses, and, without thinking about it further, I heard myself asking her if I could attend. Madame said I could participate as an observer, but only certified massage therapists were allowed to work "hands on."

My desire to study Aromatherapy was not really a snap decision. For many years I had been fascinated with the healing arts, especially health systems that emphasized natural healing techniques and time-honored cures, instead of conventional Western medicine. Even when I was only ten, I used to try to revive small dead animals with Daddy's twelve-year-old scotch! When I was in my twenties, a vegetarian diet had relieved virtually all symptoms of a crippling case of arthritis, which had threatened to end my youthful career as a dancer prematurely. Since then, I'd traveled with my own vegetable juicer, and avoided alcohol, sugar, caffeine, and meat. I'd often found myself advising friends as to how to relieve minor health and beauty problems the natural way.

As an observer of Madame Arcier's course, I watched the Aromatherapy massage technique being demonstrated and saw how restorative mixtures of essential oils could dramatically change the way people look and feel. I knew I wanted to become an Aromatherapy practitioner myself.

I returned to the States, determined to get a degree in massage therapy, so I would be eligible to work hands on in Madame's next course. A licensed therapist, who practiced in a small clinic, agreed to instruct me privately. As the training progressed, I began to treat some of the clinic's patients— one of whom I shall never forget.

I had begun using essential-oil mixtures in my treatments with gratifying results. Patients remarked that the lovely fragrances seemed to give them a more total feeling of relaxation. Then, I was asked to massage a young woman who was blind. I chose a particularly uplifting combination of juniper, basil, and lavender in my oils. As I applied this therapeutic treatment, I told her what I was trying to accomplish, and that I thought her skin and internal organs would react positively to the oils, as well as her nose. "Oh, but I lost my sense of smell in the car crash, as well as my sight," she told me.

Here was the first real challenge of Aromatherapy's effectiveness. Could I help a patient without a sense of smell with a treatment whose power came from fragrant oils? The results amazed us both. The woman continued to come to me for treatments, claiming after each one that something "special" was happening; she had more energy, her balance was better, and, most important, she felt much less depressed. Her body was able to utilize the healing and strengthening forces my treatments had set into motion; her system comprehended the revitalizing effect of the oils, even if her nose couldn't actually smell them. I now had proof of Aromatherapy's reach, and its potent impact.

After I received my massage therapy certification, I returned to London and took Micheline Arcier's course, fully hands on. Madame Arcier was an exacting teacher. She had spent forty years perfecting her massage method, and she wasn't about to give her seal of approval to any student who hadn't mastered its every nuance. She insisted that all ten of my fingers memorize each of her techniques; like a song, she said, each massage movement has a meaning. The other students and I learned to approach the human body like a finely tuned instrument; we learned to judge the response to every touch. I also discovered how Arcier's system works with the body's most subtle forces. Aromatherapy goes beyond the relaxing and stimulating effects of most massage techniques, and nudges the lymph (which cleanses and nourishes the blood) to work more efficiently, while it marshals the nerve network to balance body rhythms, improving sluggish digestion and elimination processes. Many modern problems, ranging from chronic exhaustion and overweight to skin blemishes and sinus conditions, could be relieved by Aromatherapy.

I began my own professional Aromatherapy practice in my Connecticut home, located, appropriately, on Serenity Lane. My first clients were curious members of my family and friends. I never had to advertise—Aromatherapy advertised itself. The enthusiasm of those I treated inspired others to call.

The desire to expand the influence of Aromatherapy, and to bring the healing, enhancing delight of "scentual touch" to as many as possible, has led me to write this book. I want to share my knowledge of the ways this ancient art and science of massage can relax and revitalize our modern lives, and to help others share it with those they love. Aromatherapy is not a system that only experts can practice. *You* can discover for yourself the powerful secrets of the essences—which stimulate, which relax, which can be used to dispel aches, tension, and fatigue, which can enhance beauty, in aromatic baths and teas as well as through massage. *You* can embark on this fragrant journey of the senses and learn the sorcery of scent. *You* can learn to use your fingers in conjunction with these essences to press and stroke new vitality, relaxation, and sensual awareness into others' bodies and your own. I invite my readers to discover what a joy it can be to learn this remarkable technique for getting in touch with others as well as themselves, to experience, as I have, Aromatherapy's scentual power of health, beauty, and well-being.

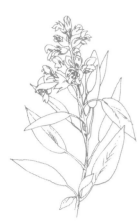

# I

# AROMATHERAPY: THE SENSUAL SCIENCE

Through massage, baths, teas, and other therapies, Aromatherapy applies essential oils to revive, to restore, to *heal* the body. Aromatherapy is part of a natural healing tradition that is more than eight thousand years old. Before the mid-nineteenth century, all remedies for chronic ailments, pain, and infectious disease were derived from plants, which were believed to have spiritual as well as curative powers. Throughout the ages, the art of natural healing was a serious science. Priests, doctors, and medicine men, from China to the Americas, brewed aromatic potions from leaves, flowers, and herbs, and used them in combination with therapeutic techniques, which included massage, or "the laying on of hands." Seductively scented oils and incense made from plants mitigated pain and also inspired pleasure in stimulating baths and perfumes, and were given to the gods as religious offerings. Though we now tend to take a skeptical view of the power of plants, reaching instead for less subtle, quicker-acting drugstore prescriptions, scientific analysis has shown that natural, time-honored herbal medicines can be remarkably effective.

## AROMATICS AND THE ANCIENTS

The history of Aromatherapy begins with Neanderthal man, who, archeologists believe, was one of the first users of plant-based medications. In 1975, a skeleton, nearly sixty thousand years old, was discovered in Iraq. Beside this ancient man, named Shanidar IV, were found concentrated de-

6

posits of pollen from yarrow, groundsel, and grape hyacinth, medicinal plants still grown and used today by Iraqi peasants. Scientists theorize that Shanidar IV was a shaman, or religious leader, and a knowledgeable botanist. Seeds from medicinal herbs and grinding slabs, the ancient pharmacologist's tool, have also been found in Central and North American excavations, dating back to 3,000 B.C.

History recorded by ancient scribes documents the therapeutic use of plants and scented oils long before the birth of Christ. In one of the oldest medical textbooks, written in 2,000 B.C., Chinese emperor Kiwang-Ti described the medical properties of opium, rhubarb, and pomegranate. Even before that, hieroglyphics tell us, Egyptians used aromatic plants for both medical and religious purposes. Plant-derived resins and perfumed oils played an important role in Egyptian funerary practices. Early embalmers mummified the dead by covering their bodies with an imported molten resin from coniferous trees. This resin suppressed bacterial activity, helping royal family members arrive in the afterworld intact. The linens, which embalmed the mummies, were soaked in frankincense and myrrh, brought back from Africa by Eighteenth Dynasty Queen Hatshepsut's expeditions. Sacred to the god of the moon, myrrh was prescribed as an anti-inflammatory agent by Egyptian priests, who were the society's healers. Myrrh was also wafted in incense burners, to intrigue the noses, and to secure the good will of the divinities. In fact, Egyptians believed aromatic medicines were effective, precisely because they had been formulated by one of the gods. But scents were also essential to the pleasures of Egyptian life. Myrrh and frankincense were combined with rosemary and thyme and shaped into perfumed cones of fat, which Egyptian men wore under their elaborate wigs. The heat of the Nile gradually melted the cones, covering faces and bodies with this organic—if slippery—form of deodorant. The pharaohs, of course, commanded the rarest perfumes—King Tut's tomb contained delicate alabaster vases filled with fragrances, which had retained their ancient aromas since 1,350 B.C.

Though the Egyptians initiated the art of extracting essences from plants by heating them in clay containers two centuries before, it was Greek alchemists who invented distillation. (Distilling essences from plants by boiling them or steaming them preserves both their fragrance and their healing properties.) Greek doctors, too, advanced the science of aromatic medications.

Dioscorides, a Greek physician, summed up man's knowledge of the use of medicinal plants in his writings; he noted, for example, that drancuculus, a plant with a stalk "spotted like a serpent's belly," checks cancer, is an abortifacient, cures gangrene, and is good for eyesight. Galen, the renowned Greek physician, was one of the world's leading herbalists. His famous textbook on the use of plants became the Western world's standard medical bible for fifteen hundred years, and was found on the bookshelves of European monasteries. Galen provided a recipe for "theraic," a medication created from a combination of 150 plants, animal parts, minerals, and even precious stones. A panacea for all ills ranging from headaches to leprosy, theraic was prescribed in France until the seventeenth century and was carried aboard seagoing vessels for hundreds of years.

Another Greek, Theophrastus, was the first true Aromatherapist. He wrote a pathfinding treatise on scent, *Concerning Odors*, in which he discussed the effect of various aromatics on thinking, feeling, and health. He also investigated the process by which we perceive odors, and the subtle relationship between taste and smell.

The Romans borrowed much medical knowledge from the Greeks, but it was the hedonistic Romans themselves who improved the ability of aromatics to delight. In Nero's palace unique silver pipes sprayed perfumes on the pleasure-loving guests. By A.D. 3, Rome had become the bathing capital of the world, with one thousand fragrant watering spots located throughout the city. Each bath had its own "unctuarium" where bathers were oiled and massaged. For Romans the scent of roses had special appeal: at one of ruthless Nero's celebrations, four million sesterces' worth of roses (about $100,000 worth) paved the city with their sweetness.

Conquests, crusades, and the growth of trade networks spread and combined the knowledge and techniques of herbalists and perfumers. Alexander's conquest of Afghanistan resulted in a fortuitous marriage of Greek and Indian medicinal lore. The Romans' far-reaching trade routes enabled them to import East Indian spices, and gum resins from Arabia, where some important new aromatic products and processes were being developed. It was the Arabians who finally perfected distillation, creating the most potent of essences. During the European Dark Ages, the Arabic world, famed for its exotic perfumes, continued to improve upon its seductive scents and magical potions. Incense, myrrh, and other species were imported from Mecca for Arabian chemists. One Yakub al-kindi of Baghdad, who lived about A.D. 850, described the distillation of musk and balsams in his *Book of Perfumes and Distillations*. Avicenna, the "Prince of Pharmacists," was the first to distill the essence of rose—an expensive process since it takes one thousand kilos of rose petals to make five hundred grams of essence. (Oil of rose now costs about thirty thousand dollars a liter.) Avicenna felt that attar of rose, a sure cure for digestive ailments, was worth the cost.

The Arab trade connections made essential oils a key ingredient in international commerce. They imported balsam from Egypt, saffron and sandalwood from India, and camphor from China. Musk was brought over the Himalayas from Tibet. The Arabs employed the new fragrances in unique ways. They mixed musk with the mortar used to build mosques, so that the sacred buildings gave off a pungent odor at noon. They used attar of rose to scent the leather gloves they sold to the European upper class.

The crusaders learned improved methods for the distillation of essences from the Arabs and brought this skill back to their own countries. By the Middle Ages apothecary guilds were established in Northern Europe, and the essential spices and oils imported from the East enhanced the quality of life, as well as the average European's chance of survival. During the Great Plague, resinous incense from pine, cypress, and cedar was burned in the streets, sickrooms, and hospitals. Perfumers who dispensed the incense apparently were untouched by the virulent disease that annihilated a large percentage of the population. Today, we have scientific proof of the antibacterial action of these natural antiseptic oils.

In the fifteenth century, essential oils continued to influence the health and happiness of Europe. Some perfumers created not only seductive scents, but lethal poisons. Catherine de Medici, about to marry the king of France, brought her perfumer with her in case she needed to dispatch a few poisoned gloves to her enemies. Aside from the occasional Machiavellian plot, essences were put to very good use to fight infections. A favorite medication, "four thieves vinegar"—a concoction of absinthe, rosemary, sage, mint, lavender, cinnamon, clove, nutmeg, garlic, and camphor macerated in red vinegar—was rubbed all over the body to keep sickness at bay.

European conquistadores discovered new medical plants during the age of exploration. The Spaniards were astounded by Montezuma's botanical gardens, which provided Aztec physicians with raw materials for medicinal formulas.

In North America, white settlers borrowed many effective herbal cures from the American natives. The Iroquois, for example, drank spruce tree tea for vitamin C, which they knew prevented scurvy. Other tribes used leatherwood and sarsaparilla as remedies; in 1708 these substances were still being used to alleviate the pain of ulcers, hemorrhoids, and cancer. Indian women had fewer deaths in childbirth than European women in the seventeenth and eighteenth centuries. They drank blue cohosh tea, which has since been found to contain caulosaponine, which provokes strong uterine contractions, ensuring easy childbirth. They also used plants, like wild ginger, a strong natural antibiotic, to protect them in childbirth.

In the mid-nineteenth century, scientific investigation into the exact effect of essential oils on bacteria in humans began in Europe and Great Britain. French researchers, for example, proved that the tuberculosis bacillus can be laid low by the essence of cloves, and that the essence of thyme in a 5 percent solution can vanquish typhus and other bacteria in less than ten minutes. Thymol, an antibacterial agent that is harmless to tissue, is used by many cosmetic houses today.

For thousands of years, then, plants—in the form of essential oils, ointments, incenses, and infusions—served not only to provide pleasure and delight, but also to wage war on disease. When the age of modern medicine dawned, however, people began to rely on the speedy action of antibiotics and other manufactured pharmaceuticals. Although "miracle drugs" have brought enormous benefits, their use led to the move away from the world of plants and to the loss of the beneficial touch of healers, not to mention the pleasures of touching and healing one another. Synthetic substances—often with unpleasant allergenic side effects—replaced natural ones, not only in medicines, but in perfumes as well. Fortunately, some astute French researchers prevented the age-old tradition of aromatic healing from being obliterated.

## THE BIRTH OF MODERN AROMATHERAPY

Rene-Maurice Gattefosse, a French chemist, founded early in this century an essential-oil house that produced oils for use in cosmetics and fragrances. One day Gattefosse burned his hand in his laboratory. Remembering that lavender was supposed to heal burns and reduce inflammation, he immediately immersed his hand in a container of pure lavender on his workbench. The burn quickly lost its redness, and began to heal. Impressed by the oil's restorative ability, Gattefosse began his research into the curative powers of essential oils. Gattefosse theorized that though the oils are externally applied, they are able to penetrate adjacent organs, because the skin is interrelated with the brain and nervous system. The nose and the skin, he said, can conduct the rejuvenating benefits of the oils to other parts of the body. He then classified the ways various essences affect the metabolism, nerves, digestive organs, and endocrine glands. It was Gattefosse, in fact, who coined the word *Aromatherapy* in 1928.

In Paris, the birthplace of modern Aromatherapy, a medical doctor, Jean Valnet, discovered Gattefosse's research. Intrigued by methods of natural healing, he began to devote most of his practice to experimenting with essential oils and recording the results. At about the same time, a charismatic biochemist, Marguerite Maury, developed a unique method of applying the penetrating oils with massage. Awarded the Prix International for her work in natural skin care, Madame Maury revealed much about the way essential oils could be used to relieve tension and improve the skin. Micheline Arcier studied and worked with Maury and Valnet; she further expanded the Aromatherapy approach to massage, and developed it as a total health system. Madame Arcier, who works closely with the medical community, believes modern medicine and age-old healing techniques can join forces to make us happier, healthier, more balanced people.

Today, Aromatherapy provides us with a contemporary version of an ancient healing art. Aromatherapy is based on the premise that the best way to prevent illness is to strengthen the body's self-defense mechanisms. Aromatherapy helps restore the harmony between body and mind, a harmony that is constantly sabotaged by the stresses of modern life and our polluted environment. In this way, Aromatherapy can positively affect the way we look, feel, and think. All of us can improve our health and loving communication with scentual massage and other time-proven Aromatherapy practices.

## HOW AROMATHERAPY WORKS

The Aromatherapy way to health and beauty includes three interrelated practices: (1) massage with essential oils; (2) baths, inhalants, and steaming; and (3) the use of herbs in cooking and infusions, or in teas. In the chapters to follow I will show you how you can make these three practices work for you. But for now let us take a brief look at the basic reasons *why* they work.

### Massage

Aromatherapy could be called the "sensual science" because it combines the nurturing and relaxing powers of touch with another very powerful sense— the sense of smell. In Aromatherapy massage, essential oils are applied to the skin and worked into the body using neuromuscular techniques that focus on the nervous system and the invisible channels of energy that Oriental doctors call the *meridians*. The massage loosens tight muscles and blocked tissues, zeroing in on central points in the energy system. As the skin responds to the massage, its nerve endings communicate with the internal organs, glands, nerves, and circulatory system. The effect may be either stimulating or calming, depending on the types of oils used and on the needs of the individual who is being massaged. The pure oils smell lovely, of course, but in Aromatherapy we use the oils for more than just aesthetic reasons. The oils are compatible with the skin's basic structure, and penetrate it layer by layer, moisturizing it, making it more supple, and stimulating the production of new cells. The actual scent of the oils, too, affects the body.

The nose contains ten million neurons that reach out and catch odor molecules; these are called olfactory receptors. They send odors to our emotional center in the brain, called the limbic system. This phenomenally active system is connected to other vital parts of the brain, those involved in controlling heart rate, blood pressure, breathing, reproductive behavior, memory, and reaction to stress. The glands, which regulate the release of hormones (and our enjoyment of sex), are also connected to this limbic system, or "smell brain." As the body is massaged with the powerful oils, each of which is selected for its unique, health-improving properties, the psychological as well as the physiological effects are astounding. The massage works on the body and brain at the same time, calming jangled nerves and stimulating the energy flow, which relieves tension and depression and eliminates toxins while building healthy tissues. An Aromatherapy massage, then, does nothing less than bring new life to the body, which means you not only look and feel but actually *become* younger.

### Baths, Inhalants, and Steaming

The Aromatherapy bath, an important adjunct to the massage, reinforces the basic rejuvenating benefits. Essential oils, added to water, stimulate the skin, relax, and energize. Inhalants, which have been used for thousands of years, can clean stuffed-up sinuses and congested chests. Finally, facial steaming deep-cleanses and moistens the face with penetrating vapors—one of the many ways Aromatherapy can be used to give you healthier, more beautiful skin.

### Teas and Herbs

Though essential oils can be taken internally, I do not recommend this potentially dangerous form of self-medication. The oils may be very pure, but they are potent, and, like any biologically active substance, can do much good if correctly used, and harm if they aren't. The use of herbs in teas and cuisine, however, is a safe and effective way to augment the benefits of a healthy diet. Using herbs as spices is as old as the art of cooking itself.

Aromatherapists value herbs not merely to enhance flavor, but also to improve your health. A variety of fresh and dried herbs can help detoxify some foods and aid in the digestion of others. Teas, which are easily assimilated, since they are diffused with large amounts of water, can work wonders for the brain, and improve organ functions. Teas are medicinal, however, and should be used in moderation.

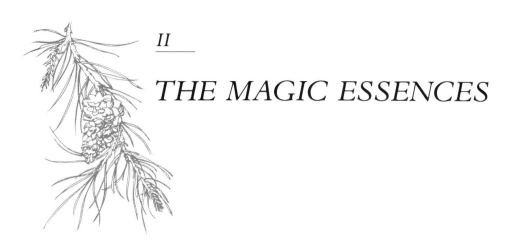

# *II*

# *THE MAGIC ESSENCES*

The most important ingredient in Aromatherapy massage and treatments is the essential oil. This pure and natural living substance is the "essence" of the plant or flower and contains the concentrated power of its vital life force.

*Oil* is actually a misleading name for these life-promoting elixirs. Aromatics are not oily at all—they are volatile essences that evaporate quickly if left exposed to the air. (That is why it is possible to use the oils in vapors as well as on the skin.) These natural organic chemicals are soluble in oil, alcohol, and a bit of water. Because the chemical compositions of the plants and flowers from which they're made are different, each oil has different actions, fragrances, and sometimes colors; patchouli oil, for example, is red, and chamomile oil is blue. You'll discover that the same complex essence may have diverse functions. Oil of bergamot, for example, has been used in the treatment of malaria, as well as in perfume. The versatile properties of cedarwood have made it an embalming agent, an aphrodisiac, an insecticide, and a basic ingredient in skin-care preparations.

The composition of essential oils allows them to penetrate the skin more effectively than ordinary vegetable oil or water. A recent experiment at the medical institute of the University of Munich, for example, demonstrated that a bath of pine-needle oil in water permeated the skin one hundred times better than water alone. Why does this happen? To begin with, essential oils are *lipophilic*, or easily mixed with fats, and the human skin is made up of fats, as well as other elements. The process of extracting the essence from the plant also reduces the size of the oil's molecules, making them smaller than the molecules that create the skin, which means the oils can enter the skin more easily. Finally, the natural chemicals that make up the essences are penetrating in themselves—which is why they should not be used undiluted on the skin without the supervision of a professional Aromatherapist. Undiluted, they may cause irritation.

In addition to their penetrating powers, essential oils also attack bacteria better than most other natural substances. They are especially valuable as antiseptics, because unlike synthetic pharmaceuticals they kill germs without harming body tissue. (Artificial antiseptics sometimes do as much harm to human cells as to the bugs they are fighting.) Scientific research has demonstrated the antiseptic effectiveness of essential oils. It has been proven that essential oils decompose and neutralize bacteria and viruses. Their fragrance does not simply cover up body odor, for example; rather, the oils through their chemical action suppress the organisms that cause body odor. Even the fragrance of essential oils can vanquish airborne germs at an amazing rate. The vapors of lemon essence will neutralize the meningitis virus in fifteen minutes and the typhus bacillus in less than an hour. The most potent essential-oil antiseptics are lemon, thyme, orange, bergamot, juniper, cloves, citronella, lavender, niaouli, peppermint, rosemary, sandalwood, eucalyptus, and Chinese anise.

## EXTRACTING THE MAGIC

Pure essential oils are obtained from the bark, roots, stalks, leaves, flowers, and resins of trees and plants. Primitive man probably chewed many of these to extract their medicinal benefits. Later, plants and flowers were pressed and made into teas, until the process of distillation was perfected. Today, extracting essences is a sophisticated process, which involves the following techniques:

> *Distillation*, or the extraction of essences by steaming, is the most popular method in use today. In this process, the plant is placed in a deep vat and steam is passed over it. The essence evaporates along with the water. This product is then cooled, and the essence is separated from the water.
> *Enfleurage* is a method used to extract flower essences, which have a tendency to disappear in distillation. Wooden frames with a glass plate on top

are covered with warm lard or suet. Petals are spread across this layer of grease and are replaced every few days until the grease is saturated with the essence. The grease is then washed with alcohol to obtain the extracts and the remaining fat is used to make soap.

*Maceration* involves soaking flowers in hot oil until their cells rupture and the oil absorbs their essence. Some essential oils are extracted in a similar way by using solvents, like petroleum, ether, and butane in extractors, which look like percolators.

*Expression* is the method by which the essence is separated from lemon, orange, and lime peels. The peel is pressed, and the liquid falls on sponges that are later squeezed to obtain the essence.

Sometimes the same plant is processed in different ways to obtain different aromatics. The orange blossom, for instance, is treated by enfleurage or solvents to produce neroli essential oil; when the fruit is ripe the skin is expressed to produce orange essence.

During a visit to one of the leading essential-oil producers in Grasse, France—the firm of Roure, Bertrand and Dupont, which has been creating outstanding aromatics since 1820—I was able to view these fascinating extraction processes. The south of France has a perfect climate for raising flowers, and has been the world's most famous center for oil production since the mid-1800s. As I walked among fragrant, shimmering pyramids of red, blue, and gold petals, past pungent bales of burlap-wrapped moss and branches with labels from every part of the world, I grasped the magic that is inherent in essential oils. As I inhaled the heady oils, bubbling and steaming into life in the vats, stills, and pressure cookers, I wouldn't have been surprised to see a vaporous genie emerge with the steam, ready to make the world smell beautiful.

## SELECTING YOUR ESSENTIAL OILS

Because the production of essential oils is a complicated art, requiring years of know-how, much equipment, and hard-to-obtain raw materials, your essences must be purchased from a reputable supply house. The only essential oils to buy are those that are *pure* and *natural*. These are more expensive than adulterated or synthetic essential oils, but worth every cent. Nothing is more costly, after all, than a product that doesn't do its job. Though it is possible to "clone" the principal components of an essence and create a synthetic that will smell much like the real one, it will not *act* the same way at all. There are components in natural essential oils that elude the chemist's identifying powers. He calls these "impurities," but it is often these unidentified substances that accomplish the oil's wonders. Do not be fooled by those who try to sell you cheaper, synthetic aromatics; they may cause allergic reactions, and they will never provide your body or nervous system with the benefits that the natural oils will.

Finding and selecting the best oils is not as easy in America as it is in countries where the use of herbs and aromatics is a respected tradition. Aromatherapy is better known in Great Britain and the European continent, where many salons and spas offer aromatic treatment and products for health and beauty. However, if you are persistent, ask questions, and teach your nose to know when a fragrance is fresh and natural, you can find top-quality essential oils in the United States, too. A resource list is included in Appendix II.

The quality and price of essential oils depend on many factors—the country that produced the plant, the abundance and quality of the crop (often dependent on climatic changes), and the way the flowers and plants are collected, stored, and processed. Like wines, essential oils have good and bad years. Most oils are expensive because a huge amount of petals or leaves is needed to produce a small amount of essence. For example, two thousand pounds of rose and jasmine petals yield a mere one pound of oil, and they must be processed very carefully, since florals, in particular, yield their superb essences reluctantly. Rose and jasmine essences are wildly expensive, yet worth the cost—there is nothing better than rose oil for facial skin.

When purchasing your essential oils, first ask if they are completely pure and natural. To check, you might ask the seller for details about where they come from, and how long he has been dealing with the supplier. Second, you will want to know how fresh the oils are. If the store has had the oils for more than six months, you should check them carefully. If they have been properly stored, they will keep for a number of years, but the only way you will know how well they have been preserved is by asking the seller, and using your nose.

After some experience with essential oils, you will develop an "essence sense." The more you use the oils, the more you will recognize each one as an individual, with its own power and potential. A fresh or well-kept oil has a lively, very characteristic odor, which you will come to recognize. Educate your nose with oils you have reason to believe are fresh and pure. Start with just three basic fragrances, like lavender, chamomile, and patchouli, sniffing one at a time, until you can recognize them without looking at the labels. Then go on to add another oil to your essence repertoire. This will keep your nose from becoming confused by too many beguiling scents.

## OIL COMBINATIONS

Most of the oils used in Aromatherapy treatments are combinations of several essential oils and "carriers," which are the vegetable oils used as a base for vital essences. When various oils are combined, the therapeutic impact of the oils is often multiplied, and different mixtures are used according to the needs of the individual. Some time-tested combinations, which I have included in Appendix I, have proved highly effective for many conditions, from insomnia and migraine to sunburn and cellulite. Making a mixture is an exciting, but exacting task. The more precise and thoughtful you are about how you combine the essential and carrier oils, the more rewarding will be the results. Complete instructions on selecting carrier oils and storing, handling, and mixing essential oils appear also in Appendix I.

## THE TWENTY-SEVEN ESSENTIAL ESSENCES

There are several hundred essential oils produced today. I have selected a limited group for the beginning Aromatherapist and give below each one's history and properties, and list some of the conditions it can treat. These basic oils are relatively easy to obtain and understand, and have proved their worth for thousands of years. They will provide the same results as harder-to-obtain essences. You may want to check the list of excellent reference books on essential oils at the back of the book for more information about the twenty-seven basics and other, rarer essences.

## BASIL

*History*: An herb that originated in Asia, basil, or "tulsi," is sacred in India, and is an important ingredient in traditional Aryuvedic medicine. The name *basil* is derived from the Greek *basilicon*, which means "a royal remedy."

*Properties*: Antidepressant; antiseptic; digestive tonic; stimulant of hormones produced by the adrenal gland.

*Can be used to treat*: Depression; fainting; mental fatigue; migraine; nausea; nervous tension.

## BAY

*History*: The leaves from the bay tree, which originated in Europe and the Americas, were used for centuries in European cuisine. Turn-of-the-century English gentlemen favored "bay rum" hair tonic—a mixture of the essence with alcohol.

*Properties:* Antiseptic; tonic; decongestant.

*Can be used to treat*: Lung conditions; colds.

## CAJEPUT

*History*: This essence comes from a tree that grows in the Philippines, Malaysia, the Moluccas, and the Celebes. The name *caje put* means "white tree."

*Properties:* Antiseptic; pain reliever; insecticide.

*Can be used to treat:* Lung congestion; neuralgia; acne.

## CEDARWOOD

*History:* From a tree that grows in America, Lebanon, southern Europe, and the Orient, cedarwood oil may have been the first essence extracted from a plant. The Egyptians used a crude method of distillation to obtain cedarwood gum, an important ingredient in their mummifying process.

*Properties:* Antiseptic; astringent; sedative; digestive stimulant; expectorant (promotes spitting); aphrodisiac.

*Can be used to treat:* Lung congestion; skin conditions such as eczema. Encourages sexual response.

## CHAMOMILE

*History:* Egyptian sages dedicated chamomile to the sun, because of its ability to reduce fever. Contains azulene, which has remarkable healing and antibacterial powers. There are two kinds of chamomile flowers: German, which is mild, and Roman, which is strong.

*Properties:* Tonic; calming agent; pain reliever; digestive stimulant; antibacterial agent.

*Can be used to treat:* Skin conditions and inflammations; nervous tension; neuralgia; digestive problems; rheumatism; insomnia.

## CINNAMON

*History:* Cinnamon trees grow in China and Ceylon. One of the oldest aromatic plants—mentioned in the Old Testament—cinnamon contains eugenol, a powerful antiseptic.

*Properties:* Antiseptic; circulatory, heart, digestive, and respiratory stimulant; antispasmodic; aphrodisiac; antivenom agent.

*Can be used to treat:* General weakness; contagious disease; muscular nerve spasms; infections; impotence; snakebites.

## CLOVE

*History*: From an evergreen tree that grows in Madagascar and the West Indies, clove, an active antiseptic, was considered a cure-all for centuries.

*Properties*: Antiseptic; mental and physical stimulant; antispasmodic; pain reliever.

*Can be used to treat*: Infections; muscular and nerve tension; general weakness. Also an excellent mouthwash and room freshener.

## CYPRESS

*History*: From the leaves and shoots of a southern European evergreen, cypress essence was a favorite aromatic of the Assyrians. Contains active healing agents.

*Properties*: Astringent; restorative agent; antispasmodic; deodorant.

*Can be used to treat*: Coughs; rheumatism; flu; wounds; muscle and nerve tension; enlarged veins.

## EUCALYPTUS

*History*: Also known as the gum tree, three hundred varieties of eucalyptus are found in southern Europe, Australia, and the American west coast. Because eucalyptus was thought to detoxify the environment, the sickly often relocated to places where the tree grew to improve their health.

*Properties*: Antiseptic; soothing agent; stimulant; insect repellent.

*Can be used to treat*: Flu; sinus problems; laryngitis; asthma; rheumatism; coughs; cuts and wounds. Also disinfects the air.

## GERANIUM

*History*: Of the seven hundred species of this flowering plant, Geranium Bourbon is the one most used by Aromatherapists. The ancients regarded geranium essence as an exceptional healing agent for wounds and fractures.

*Properties*: Tonic; stimulant of hormones from the adrenal glands; pain reliever; astringent; insect repellent.

*Can be used to treat*: Poor circulation; neuralgia; wounds; burns; mastitis, or inflammation of the breasts. Also tones the skin.

## JUNIPER

*History*: Known since antiquity for its antiseptic and diuretic powers, the juniper essence, distilled from berries, contains juniperine and camphor. The tree, or bush, grows in many countries.

*Properties*: Tonic for nervous system; digestive stimulant; diuretic.

*Can be used to treat*: Fatigue; sluggish digestion; water retention; rheumatism; sores.

## LAVENDER

*History*: A favorite aromatic of the Romans for bathing, the name comes from the Latin verb *lavare*, "to wash." The flowering plant is found in the Midi region of France and in Italy and England. Lavender grows in high altitudes: the higher the altitude, the better the quality of lavender.

*Properties*: Antispasmodic; relieves pain by calming cerebrospinal area; antiseptic; restorative; insect repellent.

*Can be used to treat*: Nervous conditions; wounds; burns; acne. Makes a good douche.

## LEMON

*History*: The Greeks called lemon *medica*, because it was imported from Medie in Asia, where it was used to perfume clothes. Now lemon is cultivated in Mediterranean countries and America. One of the most vitamin-rich essential oils, lemon contains vitamin C, carotene (a form of vitamin A), and bioflavonoids.

*Properties*: Tonic; antiseptic; diuretic; a preventive for scurvy; age retardant (prevents hardening of body tissues); insect repellent.

*Can be used to treat*: Rheumatism; gout; gastric upsets; water retention; poor skin tone. Also used in astringent skin-care preparations.

## MYRRH

*History*: From northeast Africa and Arabia, myrrh was known as *phun* in ancient Egypt and burned during the sun-worshipping ritual. Also found in the "garden of Eden" between the Tigris and Euphrates rivers.

*Properties*: Antiseptic; astringent; tonic; healing agent.

*Can be used to treat*: Infections; wounds; coughs; mouth and skin ulcers.

## NEROLI

*History*: Made from the blossoms of the bitter orange tree, neroli perfumed the gloves of Anne-Marie, Princess of Nerola, in the sixteenth century. Neroli is still used in fragrances.

*Properties*: Antidepressant; aphrodisiac; antiseptic; digestive aid; sedative.

*Can be used to treat*: Depression; insomnia; nervous tension; digestive upsets; low libido. Also used in skin preparations.

## NIAOULI

*History*: Niaouli essence, from the leaves and stems of the Melaeleuca tree, which grows in New Caledonia, contains gomenol, used in pharmaceutical preparations.

*Properties*: Antiseptic; soothing agent; pain reliever; decongestant.

*Can be used to treat*: Bronchitis; flu; coughs; sinus problems. Also a good room disinfectant.

## OLIBANUM (Incense)

*History*: An incense made from the white serum under the bark of a small tree that grows in northeast Africa and southeast Arabia, olibanum is one of the oldest aromatics. It was used by the ancients for religious ceremonies.

*Properties*: Antiseptic; blood coagulant; cleanser (causes sweating).

*Can be used to treat*: Wounds; bronchitis; asthma. Purifies polluted air.


## PATCHOULI

*History*: East Indians have used patchouli, from a small Malaysian and Indian plant, to perfume textiles for hundreds of years. The British discovered patchouli in 1820, when they imported Indian shawls impregnated with the scent.

*Properties*: Antiseptic; antidepressant; sedative; aphrodisiac.

*Can be used to treat*: Anxiety; skin conditions (acne, eczema, herpes, ulcers); "tired" skin. Also encourages sexual response.


## PEPPERMINT

*History*: Peppermint was used by the Egyptians and Israelites for its cooling effect. Hippocrates prescribed it as a stimulant and diuretic. From a small plant widely grown in temperate climates, peppermint contains menthol.

*Properties*: Stimulant for nervous system; digestive aid; antispasmodic; pain reliever; insect repellent.

*Can be used to treat*: Fatigue; indigestion; flatulence; migraine; asthma; bronchitis.


## PINE

*History*: North American Indians knew of the scurvy-preventing action of pine needles, and the antiseptic power of the bark and berries, which contain turpentine. Many varieties of pine grow in northern climates.

*Properties*: Antiseptic; diuretic; stimulant of hormones from the adrenal glands.

*Can be used to treat*: Infections; water retention; fatigue; rheumatism; gout; flu; bronchitis. Good room disinfectant.

## ROSE

*History*: One of the most adored ancient flowers, rose was known for its fragrance and healing elements. Bouquets have been found in Tutankhamen's tomb. Arab doctors were the first to use rose as a remedy in the form of "zuccar," or rose jam. Today roses are grown all over the world; the most expensive rose essence, known as rose otto, comes from Bulgaria. Rose de mai, another famous essence, is produced in Grasse.

*Properties*: Antibacterial agent; regulator of female sex organs; aphrodisiac; antidepressant; astringent; sedative; tonic for the heart, stomach, liver, and uterus.

*Can be used to treat*: Depression; poor sex drive; nausea; headache; insomnia. Also good for skin care and douching.

## ROSEMARY

*History*: Rosemary was believed by both the Greeks and the Romans to be a sacred plant with magical powers. In the Middle Ages it was burned to fumigate sickrooms. The herb is grown in the south of France, Italy, Spain, Tunisia, and America.

*Properties*: General stimulant; stimulant of hormones produced by adrenal glands; lung antiseptic; decongestant; insect repellent.

*Can be used to treat*: Fatigue; colds; flu; rheumatism; gout; skin problems (sores and burns); migraine. Also good for reducing fatty tissues.

## SAGE

*History*: The Romans called sage *herba sacra*, or "sacred herb." There are five hundred varieties of sage, which is grown everywhere, and has been used in every culture for cooking and healing. Sage clary (*salvia sclarea*) has a more attractive smell (it's minty), and is more expensive, but Sage officinalis (*sabria officinalis*) is more therapeutic.

*Properties*: Tonic; antiseptic; diuretic; regulates blood pressure and the female reproductive system.

*Can be used to treat*: Fatigue; nervousness; asthma; bronchitis; problems resulting from menopause (contains a natural plant hormone); low blood pressure. Can be used in a douche.

## SANDALWOOD

*History*: The sandalwood tree has been sacred in India since the fifth century B.C., when it was mentioned in the Nirukta, the oldest religious writing. Today the Indian government owns all sandalwood trees in order to preserve them, and they are used mostly for essence. Sandalwood is high in antiseptic alcohols.

*Properties*: Antiseptic; tonic; aphrodisiac.

*Can be used to treat*: Fatigue; bronchitis; urinary infections; impotence. Also used for fragrance.

## THYME

*History*: This ubiquitous herb was a favorite of the Egyptians, Greeks, and Romans. Since the sixteenth century, essential oil of thyme was written about in books describing pharmaceutical preparations.

*Properties*: General stimulant; antispasmodic; antiseptic; antivenom agent.

*Can be used to treat*: Fatigue; digestive problems; infectious diseases; rheumatism; skin inflammations; asthma; intestinal parasites; snakebites.

## VETIVER

*History*: An essential oil extracted from the roots of a wild grass that grows in India, Ceylon, Indonesia, Japan, and many other parts of the world, including the Caribbean and South America, vetiver's earthy aroma has long been prized for perfumes. Called "the oil of tranquility."

*Properties*: Extremely calming.

*Can be used to treat*: Anxiety; nervous tension.

## YLANG-YLANG

*History*: The flowers of a tree found in the Far East and the Philippines produce this essential oil.

*Properties*: Blood pressure regulator; sedative; antiseptic; aphrodisiac.

*Can be used to treat*: High blood pressure; intestinal infections; impotence. Widely used in fragrances.

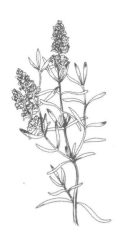

*III*

# SCENTED TOUCH: THE BASIC MASSAGE

An infant cradled in his parent's arms knows the pleasurable sensations of comfort, warmth, and security. The parental touch nourishes him and reassures him that he is loved. As a fetus in his mother's womb, touch was the first of the five senses he developed, and it is through this crucial ability to *feel* that the newborn child learns about pleasure and pain. Yet it often seems as if the sense of touch, the first we all develop, is the first to be lost as we grow older.

Touch is the sense we value least today. Most of us touch, and are touched, infrequently in the home and the workplace. We receive more sensations through our eyes and our ears than through our skin and fingertips. What we touch most often in the twentieth century are the buttons of machines. In a mechanized and electronic world, touch is a sensation we reserve for the bedroom, and lavish only on children and sexual partners. How many friends touch one another? Doctors and other health professionals touch their patients as little as possible. How many of us take the time to touch relatives, except when we greet them or say goodbye? People who aren't touched enough suffer emotional deprivation. Geriatric studies have shown that senility in the elderly is often a response to sensual starvation, and can be reversed when they are stroked and caressed. In a stress-filled, hi-tech, impersonal world, which tends to isolate us from one another, we need to touch—and be touched—in order to feel needed, content, and secure.

Massage, a therapeutic touch system, is an excellent way to put the relaxing, stimulating, and emotionally gratifying power of touch back into our lives.

## THE TECHNOLOGY OF TOUCH

Nature has custom-designed the skin and the layer beneath it to process sensation. Feeling is transmitted to the body and brain through an elaborate network of touch receptors—blood corpuscles and nerve endings—on and under the skin in the form of natural electrical charges. This highly charged network makes our sense of touch extremely sensitive. Some of the touch receptors can react when the skin has been indented only 0.0002 of an inch in a tenth of a second. Some areas of the body, such as the fingertips, palms, toes, soles, lips, tongue, and sexual areas, like the nipples, clitoris, and penis, have particularly reactive corpuscles. Hairy parts of the skin are supersensitive, too, because each hair is rooted in a follicle that is surrounded by a nerve. The downy hair, or "peach fuzz," on a woman's face is more reactive than coarse hairs, called "guard hairs," and registers a sensation when moved as little as 0.00004 of an inch. These touch receptors make it possible not only to feel, but to *hear* through the skin, which has been shown to register vibrations. The sensitivity of the skin, as well as its ability to relay the effect of touch to the rest of the body, is why massage is able to improve gland, organ, and nerve function while it relaxes the muscles and gives a positive, emotional feeling.

## AROMATHERAPY TOUCH TECHNIQUES

Massage is a science of touch, and different systems have evolved in different parts of the world. Aromatherapy, a relatively modern system, is an amalgam of four potent therapies:

*Swedish massage* uses sweeping and stroking movements to penetrate and relax the muscles. The Swedish movements in Aromatherapy are useful for delivering nourishing essential oils to the skin, loosening tense tissue, and stimulating sluggish blood circulation.

*Shiatsu*, or finger-pressure massage, is a Japanese system in which hundreds of specific points on the body, called *tsubo*, are pressed to relieve aches, tension, fatigue, and symptoms of disease. Located in the body's skin and muscular system, the tsubo function as stations along invisible routes that conduct the body's energy flow. These routes are called *meridians*. Pressing the tsubo releases the energy in the meridians when it gets blocked. According to Oriental medical philosophy, energy blockages are responsible for fatigue and illness.

*Reflexology*, like Shiatsu, zeroes in on important spots that govern the body's reflexes and glands. For example, to stimulate the thyroid, adrenals, and sexual glands, reflexologists press the pituitary point at the top of the head, which affects all glandular function. Reflexologists also believe that all the important organs have nerve endings in the feet, and that by massaging and pressing the toes, heels, and soles all the organs in the body can benefit.

*Polarity* is a method of balancing and stimulating the body's flow of energy by using its natural electrical currents in conjunction with the currents of the person doing the massage. In polarity massage the fingers of the right hand are used to stimulate and the left hand, laid flat, is used to calm.

Aromatherapists have borrowed elements from each of these effective massage systems and incorporated them into a unique touch therapy. All the benefits of the massage are multiplied by the addition of the rejuvenating essential oils.

## WHAT THE AROMATHERAPY MASSAGE SYSTEM DOES

During an Aromatherapy massage you will be using your sense of touch to diagnose the general physiological condition of your massage partner, to stimulate or calm his nervous system, and to improve the function of his all-important lymphatic system, which keeps the body free of damaging toxins and affects the energy level and general health.

### AROMATHERAPY DIAGNOSIS

In Aromatherapy your sense of touch is used to analyze the texture of your massage partner's skin and its underlying tissue. With experience, your fingers will be able to discern whether the tissues are spongy (indicating water retention), whether the muscles are tight, whether the skin is dry and scaly, oily or congested. Diagnosis will tell you which techniques and oils will be most effective for the person you are massaging. Your probing touch will discover knotted fibers and tight muscles, which you can then begin to relax. Even mental tension can be felt by touching your partner's head perceptively. As you practice Aromatherapy you will develop your natural touch intuitions, and will learn much about your partner's body as well as your own—because as you are touching, *you* are also being touched. In the section "Pre-Massage Diagnosis" (on page 44) and in my step-by-step instructions for massage technique, you will learn just how to do "fingertip diagnosis."

### LIBERATING THE LYMPH

One of Aromatherapy's most important tasks is to improve the function of the lymphatic system. Few people are familiar with the all-important lymph, or realize how vital it is to energy and health. Lymph is a colorless fluid that flows through the body along with the blood. Made up of water and waste products, lymph is absorbed by the tissues into a map of tiny, thread-like capillaries that cover the body. (See Diagram 1.) These capillaries act like tiny conduits, running into larger vessels, which in turn empty into still larger lymphatic glands, or nodes. The lymph nodes filter the lymph as it passes through, purifying it, and producing antibodies, antitoxins, and cells that process the lymph itself. After this cleansing and regenerative process, the lymph travels back into the bloodstream via two major veins in the neck. Unlike blood, which is pumped by the heart, lymph has no natural pump— our own activity keeps it moving from one part of the body to another. Sedentary people who suffer from tension and exhaustion and eat a diet high in refined foods, meat, and other concentrated proteins may develop blocked lymph nodes. When the lymph stops flowing freely, lymphatic tissue, like the tonsils, can become inflamed and swell, making you feel exhausted or sick. Aromatherapy massage is especially designed to liberate blocked lymph, or get it moving again; regular Aromatherapy treatments can prevent lymph blockages from occurring in the first place.

People whose bodies are *toxic*, or polluted with poisons, due to smoking, drinking, drug-taking, poor diets, or exposure to chemicals in air or water,

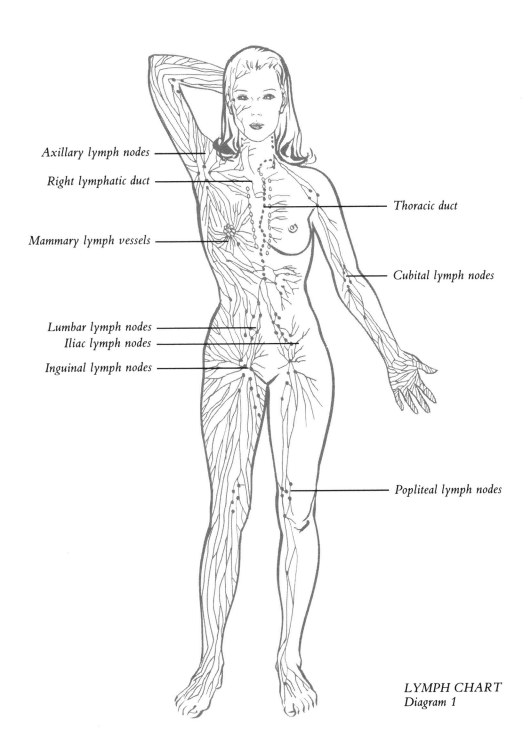

Axillary lymph nodes

Right lymphatic duct

Mammary lymph vessels

Lumbar lymph nodes

Iliac lymph nodes

Inguinal lymph nodes

Thoracic duct

Cubital lymph nodes

Popliteal lymph nodes

*LYMPH CHART*
*Diagram 1*

should be massaged very carefully, and treated over a period of time to avoid sending a rush of poisoned lymph into their systems, which can make them very ill. In the section on step-by-step massage technique (page 50), I will explain how to tell if your massage partner's lymph is blocked, and how to liberate it safely.

### BALANCING THE NERVOUS SYSTEM

The nervous system is a complex network of sensitive nerves that runs down the back of the neck and spine. Nerves communicate messages from the brain to all the other organs, via an electrical "charge," which is produced by natural chemicals in the nerve cells themselves. The nerves form clusters, or ganglia, along the spine, and these clusters have a tendency to knot up into tight bunches. In Aromatherapy massage we relax these "bundles of nerves" and decongest them by pressing and moving them in specific ways with our fingers. In the process of balancing the nerves, we also stimulate the body's organs, because relaxed nerves send brain messages more effectively. An important principle to remember is that because of the way the nervous system is structured—crossing from one side of the spinal cord to the other—sensations on the left side of the body are often coming from the right side of the brain, and vice versa. What this means is that you will often massage one side of the body to obtain a specific result on the other; for example, to ease a pain in the right side of the head, you can massage the left shoulder.

## THE IMPORTANCE OF SCENT

An important difference between Aromatherapy and other massage systems is that an Aromatherapy treatment involves the sense of smell as well as the sence of touch. While your fingers are massaging away aches and pains, and revitalizing the health of all the organs, the essential oils are stimulating and calming the body and brain.

Smells take a direct, physical route to the brain because they employ nerve cells as transmitters and receivers. Odors travel directly through the olfactory

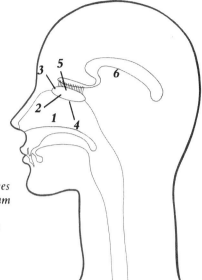

1. *Air containing odor molecules passes bony turbinates*
2. *Odor molecules are picked up by hairlike odor receptors called cilia*
3. *The cilia carry the smell message to the olfactory nerves*
4. *The message goes to the base of the olfactory epithelium*
5. *Odor interpretation begins*
6. *The interpretation is routed through the limbic system to the brain*

*SENSE OF SMELL*
*Diagram 2*

system in the nose and the front part of the head into the limbic area of the brain, which processes smell. (See Diagram 2.) *This part of the brain is also the seat of learning, memory, and emotions.* For this reason, the effortless and automatic sense of smell can trigger powerful emotions and provide vivid reminders of people and places. The smell of chocolate chip cookies, for example, can call to mind the loving grandmother who used to bake them.

The discovery that the perception of odors can have a major impact on thinking and feeling has prompted new and vigorous research into the whys and wherefores of the sense of smell. Scientists at Yale University, the Monell Institute of Chemical Senses, and Duke University are working to find out how the sense of smell affects the way we live and function. These researchers have shown, for example, that we can have a physiological response to odor: a recent experiment at Duke University's medical school revealed that when a person smells a food to which he is allergic, such as chocolate, a natural biochemical, called a *histamine*, which is secreted during allergic reactions, immediately rises in the blood.

The limbic system also has an intimate relationship with the hypothalamus, the part of the brain that communicates with the sex glands. Without this hookup between scent and sex, Earth would be a lonely planet! The chemical messenger of scent that acts as a turn-on is called a pheromone. Pheromones are an invitation to mate, especially for animals and insects; they are excreted in urine, by skin glands, and in vaginal secretions and saliva. Heady perfumes containing sexually stimulating essential oils like sandalwood, patchouli, and ylang-ylang act as pheromones for humans. When used in Aromatherapy treatments, these scents work on brain receptors to activate the sexual glands.

Essential oils, then, can improve your health, your moods, and even your relationships; the smell of lavender is calming, basil uplifting, and ylang-ylang exciting. An appropriate blend of scented oils used in an Aromatherapy treatment augments the effects of your hands and fingers.

## AROMATHERAPY POWER

Learning Aromatherapy will provide you with a powerful skill that will enhance your life and the lives of others. The first few massages you give will be a learning experience and, like any new adventure into the unknown, will be exciting and somewhat frightening.

Soon after I returned to the United States with my certification from Madame Arcier, I received a call from a dear friend. Her husband was dying of a virulent form of cancer, and she had just started a new business. From the sound of Wendy's voice on the phone, I could tell she was desperately tired, tense, and in a state of despair. I suggested that I give her an Aromatherapy treatment.

My friend was only the third person I had treated on my new massage table. I was apprehensive, since her problems were severe, and I was still a novice Aromatherapist. Could I really be helpful to someone in such a dire situation? Once my friend was lying face down, however, covered with clean sheets and towels, I began to feel more confident. I realized then that when you take the power of touch seriously, and believe in your ability to help, you lose your self-doubts and the process takes over.

Wendy's body was a major challenge to my fledgling technique. She was tense from head to toe, and holding fluid in her buttocks and legs, which made them feel spongy and lumpy. I was alarmed to see that she had bruises on her legs the diameter of oranges. Tension had so taxed her energy-supplying adrenal glands that they had used up her supply of vitamin C, which the adrenals need in order to function. The adrenals had then pulled vitamin C away from other areas that use it for such functions as maintaining the shape and structure of blood capillaries; this is why she was bruised.

I started out by giving Wendy light, soothing treatments with essential oils containing lavender and geranium; soon we were able to move on to more stimulating methods, using juniper and cypress oils to help her water-retention problem. She began to improve, and then her husband died. After several weeks of grieving, she called again, anxious to resume our massages. Her tissues had tightened up because of the gap in treatments, but she had maintained most of the fluid loss I had begun to achieve before her husband's death. At the end of the treatment she sat up on the table, hugged me, and said, "If it hadn't been for these Aromatherapy treatments I never could have pulled myself through these last three months. Your massage has brought me out of my overwrought mind and back to my own body. Thanks to Aromatherapy, I know I am still here, and still me."

These words made me think long and hard about the responsibility of touching another person's body. Aromatherapy is a revitalizing system that should make positive changes in your massage partner's health and the way he feels about himself. But it is also a potent system, and care must be taken to use it effectively. Begin with the idea that your goal is to do what is best for the person who trustingly surrenders himself to your touch. If you maintain this selfless, giving attitude, you can massage those people closest to you—parent, child, husband, or lover—without ever feeling embarrassed, prejudiced, or insecure. No matter whose body it is, treat it with reverence.

With the power of Aromatherapy in mind, you will want to prepare your massage partner and yourself—psychologically as well as physically—for the experience. During a massage there is an exchange of energy between the giver and the receiver. The expression "thoughts are things" applies to massage because touch becomes a tangible form of communication between you and your massage partner. The person giving the massage must be as balanced, centered, and calm as possible in order to balance, center, and calm the person he is massaging. Your massage partner should be encouraged by your attitude, as well as your words, to relax and let go so that the combination of touch technique and therapeutic fragrance can work its miracles.

Try to spend a few moments alone before giving a massage. Visualize yourself bathed in a benevolent light of a soft color; breathe deeply and rhythmically. Then approach your massage partner with a warm and giving spirit. Encourage your partner to breathe deeply, too, and to leave tension and negativity behind as you journey together into the blissful state of complete relaxation.

## MASSAGE PRELIMINARIES

Here are some important suggestions for getting yourself and your massage atmosphere and equipment ready for the treatment; they are not difficult to follow and will enhance the experience and result of Aromatherapy:

· *The room* where you give the massage should provide a retreat from the real world and its disrupting tensions. It should be warm or cool enough to be comfortable to the bare skin. Eliminate all possible noise, except perhaps for soothing music, such as a harp or flute concert, or a record of sea sounds. Music is optional; some Aromatherapists feel it distracts the person being massaged and prevents him from focusing inward and fully experiencing what is happening to his body. Take the telephone off the hook, or put on your answering machine if you have one. Once a treatment begins, the jangle of a phone and other interruptions can destroy the concentrated mood you want to create and maintain.
· *A professional massage table, bed, or even the floor* is a good base for massage. A massage table, of course, is preferable, because it provides the firmest, most comfortable base, as well as a cushioned opening where the face can rest comfortably when your massage partner is lying on his stomach. The height of the table is very important. Ideally, the table's top should reach

the flat of your hand when your arm is down at your side and fully extended. This height enables you to apply appropriate pressure without any strain. Leaning over a bed can be hard on your back and, unless the mattress is super firm, it will not adequately support the body on which you are working. Inserting a board under the mattress will help make it firmer. Shiatsu practitioners use the floor as a massage base, though you may find this angle and hard surface too tough on the back and the knees. Whatever your massage base, it must be totally comfortable and aesthetically appealing. The surface should be well padded, and covered with sheets and/or toweling. I use giant-sized beach towels in soothing pastels. Your massage partner should be able to relax completely, which is never possible if he feels uncomfortable.

· *Fragrance in the air* will reinforce the scent message of the essential oils. Pouring a small amount of pure essence onto a unit especially designed to heat it is the most effective way to create a fragrant atmosphere. Specialty stores that sell fragrance and bath products often carry rings made especially to hold scented oils and liquid essences that can be placed on top of a lighted bulb, as well as small warming dishes, heated underneath by a candle or from within by a low electric current. You can also use a small fondue pot. Make sure you use a pure, natural essence in your warming unit, and not a synthetic that smells like the real thing; the synthetic won't have the same physiological or psychological impact.

· *Your massage oils* should be pre-mixed (see the section "Mixing the Oils" in Appendix I) and placed at the upper left of the spot where you are standing or kneeling. This way they will be within easy reach and you won't have to contort yourself to pick them up, nor will you be forced to take your hands away from your massage partner for too long an interval. Put the bottles of oil on a surface that won't be damaged by a drippy bottle, such as a china or hard plastic dish.

· *Your hands must be clean.* Wash them well with mild soap and warm water. If your hands are cold, hold them under hot water until they feel warmer— at least normal skin temperature. A cold hand can shock a warm back, even in summer.

· *Your nails should be short*—as short as your vanity allows. A scratchy nail

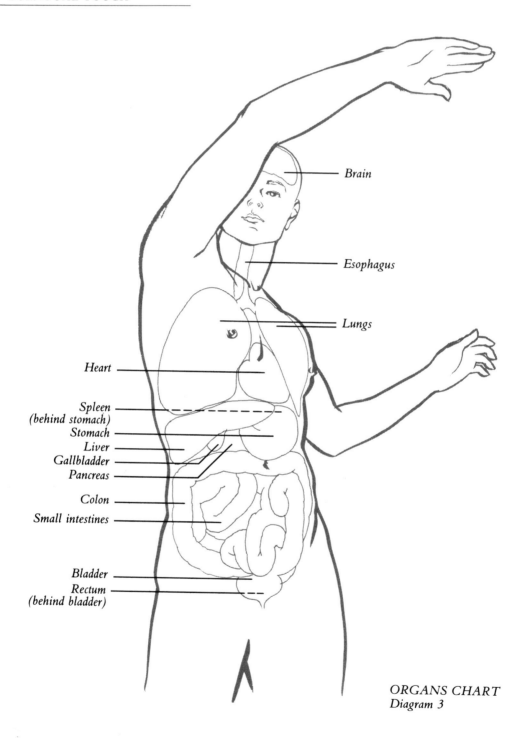

Brain

Esophagus

Lungs

Heart

Spleen
(behind stomach)
Stomach
Liver
Gallbladder
Pancreas

Colon
Small intestines

Bladder
Rectum
(behind bladder)

ORGANS CHART
Diagram 3

can ruin even the most loving touch. Run the ends of your fingers over your own skin; if you can detect the presence of a nail, your nails are too long. Ironically, the essential oils stimulate nail growth and may give some brittle-nailed ladies the talons they've always longed for; but if you're a serious Aromatherapist, you have to keep them short. (Another benefit of the essential oils is that they will make your hands look and feel smoother and younger if you treat yourself and others with them on a regular basis.)

• *Wear loose and comfortable clothes*, but not so loose as to get in your way. I like to wear pants with an elasticized waist and a loose shirt when I'm giving a massage. You will warm up as you work, so don't overdress, even in cold weather. Massage is a form of exercise! Your shoes should be light, supportive, and comfortable, like gum-soled canvas shoes.

## STUDYING THE BODY

Massage is a physiological science that requires at least a minimal working knowledge of anatomy. Diagram 3 shows you the location of the major organs of the body.

You will also need an understanding of the relationship between the nerves that are located along the spine and the body's organs. Before you begin to massage, and during your first treatments, study Diagram 4, which shows the different sections of the spine and how they relate to the rest of the body. This knowledge will improve your technique and increase your confidence.

Aromatherapy, like reflexology, divides the body into four major zones, named after the different sections of the spine:

C—Cervical (the neck area)
D—Dorsal (mid to upper back area)
L—Lumbar (mid to lower back area)
S—Sacral (lower back area)

Each of these four sections contains vertebrae, or smaller sections, to which numbers are assigned; it is easy to count down the spine and learn the zones, as well as which parts of the body they govern. Here is a list of the zones and their corresponding organs. Keep this section handy until you learn the zones by heart:

C1—Head, scalp, brain, bones of face, pituitary gland, inner ear (called "Atlas")

C2—Optic and auditory nerves, eye, forehead, mastoid bone (a projection behind the ear), tongue (called "Axis")

C3—Trigeminal nerve (through which you "sense" odors), cheeks, outer ear

C4—Nose, lips, mouth, eustachian tubes (tube between the middle ear and the throat)

C5—Vocal cords, larynx, pharynx, neck glands

C6—Neck and shoulder muscles, tonsils

C7—Thyroid gland, arm

C8—Arm (not connected to a vertebra)

D1—Esophagus, windpipe (trachea), lower arm

D2—Heart

D3—Lungs, bronchial tubes, chest, breasts

D4—Gallbladder

D5—Solar plexus, liver

D6—Stomach

D7—Pancreas, first section of small intestine (duodenum)

D8—Spleen, diaphragm

D9—Adrenal glands

D10—Kidneys

D11—Kidneys, ureter (one of tubes conveying urine from kidney to bladder)

D12—Small intestine, fallopian tubes

L1—Large intestine, colon (last section of large intestine)

L2—Appendix, abdomen, upper leg

L3—Ovaries, uterus, testes, bladder, knee

L4—Prostate gland, lower back muscles, sciatic nerve (in the hip)

L5—Lower leg, ankle, feet, toes, arches

S—Coccygeal gland (near tip of coccyx bone at end of the spine), external genitalia, rectum

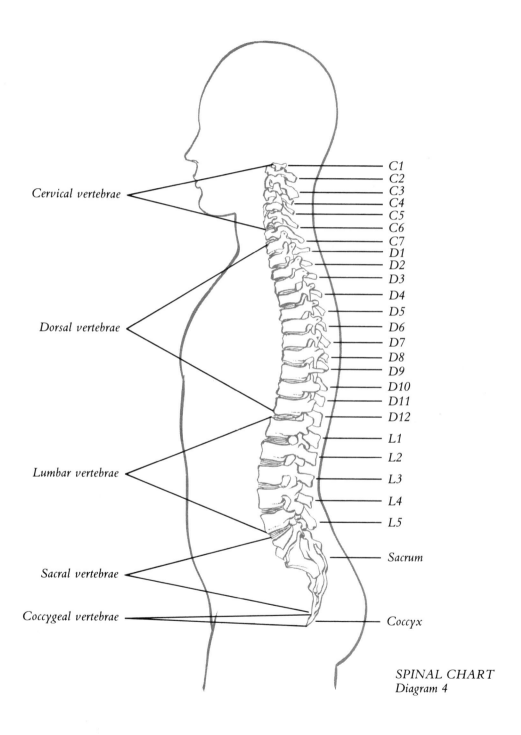

Cervical vertebrae

Dorsal vertebrae

Lumbar vertebrae

Sacral vertebrae

Coccygeal vertebrae

C1
C2
C3
C4
C5
C6
C7
D1
D2
D3
D4
D5
D6
D7
D8
D9
D10
D11
D12
L1
L2
L3
L4
L5

Sacrum

Coccyx

**SPINAL CHART**
*Diagram 4*

Diagram 5 shows the direction of the muscle fibers located within various muscle groups and their underlying bony structure. During the massage you will work either with or against the grain of the muscle fiber.

## _____ PRE-MASSAGE DIAGNOSIS _____

Before you actually begin to massage, you should have some idea of your massage partner's general physiological condition. Professional Aroma-therapists invite a new client for a consultation before beginning a series of treatments. They ask questions like: Why have you come for an Aroma-therapy treatment? Do you have any specific complaints? Are you married? Have you had any children? Did you have problems during pregnancy and childbirth? The Aromatherapist tries to get a picture of the client's life-style—diet, exercise, work, and sleep habits—and to find out if there is an unusual medical history—any accidents, broken bones, operations, or chronic illnesses.

Ideally, your first massage partners are cooperative friends or family members; you will probably know them well, and may not want or need to build up a dossier of personal information. You should, however, be aware of any particularly weak or vulnerable areas in their bodies, such as a spinal abnormality, or a shoulder that easily goes out. Ask your partner about problematic areas, and if they exist proceed with extra care when you work on them.

People communicate much about their physical and mental states by the way they walk and talk. Be alert to your massage partner's messages. Nervous, tense people speak and move quickly with abrupt gestures. A fatigued or anemic person may have very little energy at all, may speak slowly, and may have trouble organizing his thoughts. Even before your massage partner undresses, his general condition should be apparent, and let you know whether he needs a calming essence like lavender, or an uplifting one like juniper. (See the recipe section in Appendix I for mixtures for specific conditions.)

Once your massage partner has undressed and is ready for treatment, perform a quick skin analysis with your eyes, and by running your hands

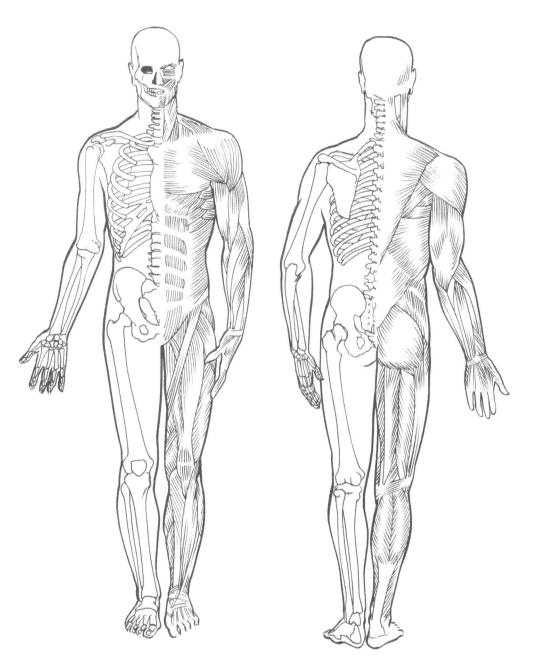

*MUSCLE/BONE CHART*
*Diagram 5*

lightly over his back, arms, and legs. Look for these basic signs:

· Skin color reveals much about your massage partner. Pale skin can signify anemia and/or low blood pressure. Flushed facial skin signals high blood pressure, and yellowish, sallow skin may mean toxicity. When you are working on your partner, take note of areas that become reddened and blotched; this discoloration can indicate trouble in corresponding organs. For example, redness in the upper back area can be a sign of heart congestion. Don't jump to hasty conclusions, however; if your partner is digesting a big meal eaten too close to massage time, it may appear as if there is a strain in the heart region. As a matter of fact, neither you nor your partner should enter the massage experience directly after a meal. Allow at least an hour between dining and massage. If you see a repeated discoloration of an area of the skin relating to a particular organ (see Diagram 7 on page 83 for the relationship between the areas of the body and major organs), you should suggest that your massage partner have a medical checkup.

· Pale, thin skin that freckles (redhead skin) should be treated with a light touch and nourishing oils. Combine 2 ounces of almond oil and 2 ounces of avocado oil; then add 8 drops of lavender and 4 drops of rose or geranium. (Before you actually mix this recipe or any of the others that follow, be sure to consult Appendix I for complete instructions regarding the selection of carrier oils and the handling and mixing of essential oils.)

· Dehydrated skin lines easily, feels dry, and may be rough or scaly. This kind of skin soaks up oil thirstily, and needs it. Try 4 ounces of sesame or soy oil with 6 drops of lavender, 4 drops of sandalwood, and 2 drops of patchouli added.

· Oily skin is most evident on the face, where oily patches can be seen on the nose, chin, and forehead. The back may also have some acne blemishes because the oil glands are blocked. This type of skin should be treated with a light formula, such as 4 ounces of safflower or sunflower oil with 6 drops of lavender, 3 drops of chamomile, and 3 drops of eucalyptus or niaouli added.

There are other indications of your massage partner's health for you to consider during your pre-treatment diagnosis:

- Cold hands and feet may mean poor circulation. A warming formula will be helpful, such as 6 drops of lavender, 4 drops of rosemary, and 2 drops of vetiver in 4 ounces of soy oil.
- Spongy tissue, which doesn't spring back quickly when you press your finger into it, means that fluid is being retained. This is a sign that the lymph system may not be working as well as it should. Tension can also cause water to be held in the tissues. Aromatherapy massage, with its relaxing, lymph-liberating technique, can help the body release stored-up fluid, especially if you treat it with a formula of 6 drops of lavender, 4 drops of juniper, and 2 drops of rosemary in 4 ounces of soy oil.
- Knotted muscle fiber is obvious and can be felt with a light touch. It is hard and "ropey." The ropey quality can be perceptibly reduced in a matter of minutes with massage using relaxing essences. Try a formula of 6 drops of lavender and 6 drops of basil or marjoram in 4 ounces of soy oil.
- Tension makes itself known in hard, congested areas on the upper back, neck, and buttocks. The tense partner will benefit from calming oils. Try a formula such as 6 drops of lavender, 4 drops of chamomile, and 2 drops of vetiver in 4 ounces of soy oil.
- Nervous, jumpy partners will find it hard to relax and lie still, and their muscles may seem to pull away from your touch. They can be calmed all over with an easygoing technique using the tension formula noted above. Movements should be slow and gentle until you gain their confidence and they begin to relax, at which point you can increase the speed and intensity of your movements. In addition, you can put a drop of vetiver in your palm, rub gently over your hand to spread it, and place your hand on a jumpy partner's diaphragm (the most sensitive nerve center of the body, just under the breast bone) to lull your partner into relaxing.

## WHEN NOT TO MASSAGE

The pleasurable benefits of Aromatherapy are so far-reaching, it is tempting to think that it will be good for everyone, and cure every problem. Not so; there are serious medical conditions that make massage prohibitive. The sick patient should definitely be left in the hands of a professional doctor. If your massage partner has, or even *seems* to have, any of the following conditions, postpone your treatment:

- Cancer
- Heart condition
- Recent serious operation
- Open wound
- Fever
- A bacterial or viral infection, such as pneumonia or flu
- Nausea

Aromatherapy stimulates the flow of blood and lymph; though this process initiates cleansing, it can also raise a temperature or spread infection. Once your partner has been cured, however, the restorative oils and touch technique can help to rebuild vitality and healthy tissues.

## _____ MAKING MASSAGE COMFORTABLE _____

Here are some important pointers for making the Aromatherapy experience more comfortable—both physically and emotionally—for you and your partner:

- Ask your massage partner to undress completely. He should be nude, so that your hands will be able to flow freely over his bare skin without obstruction. Modest people may prefer to keep on underwear, which can be rolled down during the treatment. Because your partner's skin is bare, warmth is imperative. Even in summer a sheet or large towel should cover the areas of the body you aren't working on. The towel also gives the shy person some camouflage, and makes him feel more secure. In the winter, a fluffy, washable blanket should be kept handy in case the room becomes chilly; this can be rolled up or down along with the sheets and towels.
- Your massage partner should lie face down with his arms at his sides, or, if you are using a massage table, his arms may hang down over it. As he lies down you should cover him completely with the oversized towel or sheet, which you then neatly fold back just far enough to expose the top half of his buttocks.

· You should be standing (or kneeling) to the upper left of your massage partner. (You will be working mostly from the left, except when massaging the hands and feet.) As you work try to divide your weight equally and to bring energy from your body into your hands and arms. This will protect your back, and your arms and hands will become less tired. Think of moving from your hips, not your shoulders.

· Place a small chair or stool at the upper end of the massage area, so that you can sit comfortably when working on the hands and face. (Unless, of course, you're working on the floor.)

· If your partner has a tight back, a small pillow properly placed should relieve his tension. When he is on his stomach, place the pillow under the groin. When he is on his back, the pillow should go under the knees. Correct pillow positioning can vary according to individual needs; ask your partner to tell you when he feels it is in the right spot.

· Aromatherapy massage may touch on tender spots—and tenderness can tell you much about the body's condition—but it is not a technique that is meant to be painful. If it is, *stop!*

· Discourage conversation. It may be tempting to chat and gossip in this intimate situation, but talking will impede your partner's complete relaxation. However, if he seems to have the need to get a weighty secret off his chest, the opening-up process of the massage will encourage him to do so. In that case, let him talk it out, and then try to bring him back to calming silence. Don't be surprised if a badly stressed partner begins to cry during the massage. You are touching important nerve release centers that can prompt a range of emotions, from giggles to tears. Some people drift off into a deep sleep. You may find this behavior a little unnerving; relax, and remember that emotional release is a benefit of the Aromatherapy experience.

## ___ THE MASSAGE OIL ___

Depending upon your massage partner's mood, health, and physical condition, Aromatherapy provides a host of oil formulas from which to choose. A preceding section, "Pre-Massage Diagnosis," provided formulas for specific skin types, as well as specific emotional or physical conditions. In addition, Appendix I provides a complete collection of oil formulas suitable for body and face massage.

When you are just beginning to practice Aromatherapy, you may want to start with a simple-to-make and very effective basic body oil combining 4 ounces of soy oil with 12 drops of lavender. A face oil to which most facial skin responds well is 4 ounces of sesame oil with 8 drops of chamomile. Complete instructions on how to mix the oils appear in the recipe section at the back of the book.

The most effective way to anoint your massage partner with oil is to pour about a teaspoon of the mixture you've selected into the *center* of your palm, rub your hands lightly together, and spread the oil on the body with both hands, covering only the area you intend to work on. *Never* pour the oil directly on the body; if it is cool, it will give the skin an unnerving shock. And don't pour the oil into your fingers; it will start dribbling out before you get it on the body. The oil poured into your palm, rubbed in your hands, and spread on the body will absorb your magnetic energy as it passes through your hands. Don't worry if you haven't yet been able to find the pure essential oils necessary to mix your own blend. There are good commercial massage oils, stocked by all health food stores and some pharmacies; many of these contain pure essences. These will do until you can find or order high-quality essential oils.

## STEP-BY-STEP MASSAGE TECHNIQUE

You are now ready to begin your adventure into scented touch. Be sure to follow my directions carefully. And remember that a strongly positive attitude will help give energy to both you and your massage partner, even one who is burdened with negative thoughts and feelings.

The basic massage consists of forty-three movements that cover all parts of the body. They are safe techniques and, with a little practice, will be easy to master. You may want to learn them by reading the directions carefully, and practicing on an imaginary body, much as a pianist practices on an imaginary keyboard, before you invite your first partner for a treatment. Though the directions will instruct you to cover your partner's body, the illustrations have been done without covering to make them clearer. To cover or not depends on the wishes and comfort of your massage partner.

To begin with, your massage partner should be lying face down, completely covered with a towel or sheet; the arms may be straight at the sides or hanging over the table. Uncover the body as you start to work.

### 1. Establishing Connection

This combination of movements is meant to relax your massage partner and establish your connection. It is done with dry hands. Cup your left hand around the base of the skull (the occipital bone) and keep it there (see Illustration III-1) as you do the following:

a. Rest your flat right hand in a horizontal position between the shoulders (D5, see Diagram 4 and its analysis on page 43) and count to twenty; then lift hand.

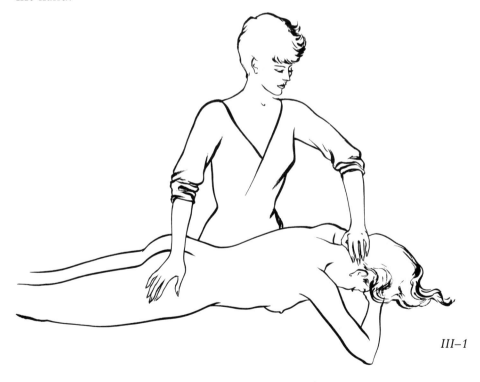

III-1

b. Rest your flat right hand between the bottom of the shoulder blades (D10, see page 43) and count to twenty; then lift hand.

c. Rest your flat right hand on the mid-back, just above the waist (L2 and L3, see page 43), and count to twenty; then lift hand.

d. Place the right hand high on the right buttock (iliac crest) and push gently. (See Illustration III–1.) Hold for twenty counts. Repeat on the left buttock. Lift the right hand and pause for a moment, while you keep your left hand on his head. This gives your massage partner an exciting feeling of anticipation for what's coming next.

### 2. *Massaging the Base of the Skull*

Remove your left hand from the base of the skull and gently massage the same area with the right hand. Use your thumb on the left side, and your fingers on the right, pulling the two sides together. This movement familiarizes you with the shape of the bottom of the occipital bone (skull bone) and prepares you for the next movement.

### 3. *Pressing the Base of the Skull*

Hold the right side of the head with the left hand and, with the thumb of your right hand, press along the base of the left side of the skull until you reach the slight hollow that divides the head. Then hold the left side of the head in your left hand and, using the third finger of the right hand, press along the base of the right side of the skull until you reach the division again. The presses should begin about one inch in from the ear. (See Illustration III–2.) The pressure should be strong enough so that your partner really feels it, but it should not be painful. Due to tension and congestion, some people are very tender in this area, so go gently at first, increasing the pressure if your partner can tolerate it. You are working in an area that communicates with the brain, pituitary gland, inner ear, and optic and auditory systems. You will be amazed to discover how different heads can be—it's enough to make you want to study phrenology! Repeat this movement three times on both sides.

### 4. *Sweeping the Skull*

Sweep your fingers over the top of the head and through the hair, starting at the base of the skull. Carry the motion all the way to the ends of the hair,

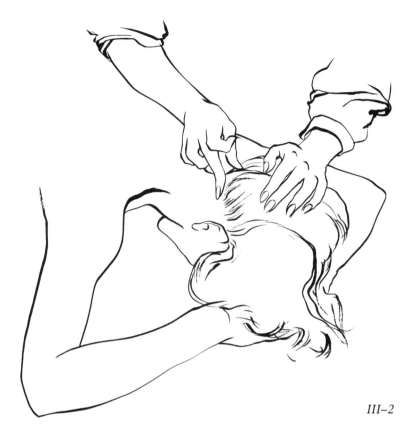

*III–2*

giving your hand a little flick at the end of each sweep. This stimulates the cranial nerves and neutralizes negative electrical charges from the body.

### 5. *Stroking on the Oil*

You are now ready to begin stroking on the essential oil. Pour the massage oil into the palm of your hand. (A teaspoonful should be enough for the upper back, but if your partner's skin is very dry, two applications may be needed. The way the skin absorbs the oil is a barometer of its condition. Dry or dehydrated skin absorbs oil more rapidly than oily skin.) Using both hands, stroke on the oil from the tailbone to the neck and over the shoulders. Then begin to stroke with a sweeping motion from bottom to top; this is called "effleurage." Place your hands together at the bottom of the spine, fingers pointing toward the head. Sweep up to the neck, then out over the

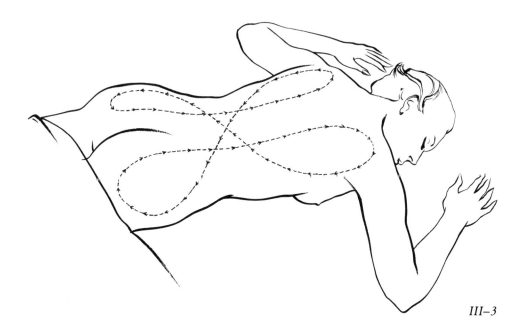

*III–3*

shoulder. Come down to mid-back, where your hands cross, and then sweep around each buttock, bringing your hands together again at the base of the spine, where the movement starts again. Repeat six times. (See Illustration III–3.) This is the first big movement you are using in the treatment; make it authoritative and enjoyable. Let your hands relax and make flexible curves around and over the contours of the body; keep your hands flat as they make the curves.

### 6. *Waking Up the Nerves Along the Spine*

You are now about to approach the thirty-one nerves that originate from the spinal cord, and the chain of ganglia (nerve clusters) that make up the sympathetic nervous system. This sounds awesome, and it is. However, keep in mind that, though our every movement and sensation is affected by our spinal nerves, they are less fragile than you would think.

For the first mvement that begins to "wake up" the spinal nerve area you will use only your thumbs. Place them at the bottom of the spine with the tips touching. Now press in with the thumbs together up the right side

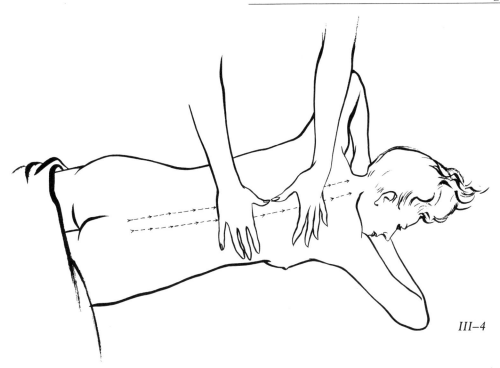

III–4

of the spine all the way to the neck; slide the thumbs and press in about every two inches. (See Illustration III–4.) Keep your thumbs on the back as you slide up and press in. Press in firmly but not too deeply. Repeat this series of presses on the left side of the spine. Do both sides three times. Never press directly on the spinal bone during this movement, or at any time during the massage.

### 7. *Sliding the Thumbs Up the Spine*

With your thumbs tip to tip (as they were in the presses in Movement 6), start at the base of the spine on the right side, and slide them up to the neck. Make three of these sweeps, then repeat three times on the left side of the spine. As you sweep, press with your thumbs and relax your hands so they slide lightly along the back.

### 8. *Decongesting the Back Tissue*

The tissue on the back, including the top skin and several layers of nerves, fat, and underlying fluid, often becomes tight and congested with tension and fatigue. You are going to relieve this congestion by picking up the skin between your two hands. Begin just above the buttocks and continue all over the back up to the neck and the top of the shoulders. Scoop up the skin, going in as deeply as you can. As you scoop, as if you were scooping up water, your fingers roll in together and touch, as you turn your hands inward. (See Illustration III–5.) You might want to practice this technique on your own thighs, especially if you want to tone them. Even if your massage partner wonders what in the world you are doing to his back, he should enjoy the sensation. Repeat three times, lifting the tissue all over the back.

### 9. Raking the Back

Beginning at the base of the spine on the partner's right side, poise the tips of the fingers of both hands at the edge of the spinal column pointing toward the table, and slide them over the back and down to the massage table or floor; the thumbs follow the fingers. (See Illustration III–6.) This "raking"

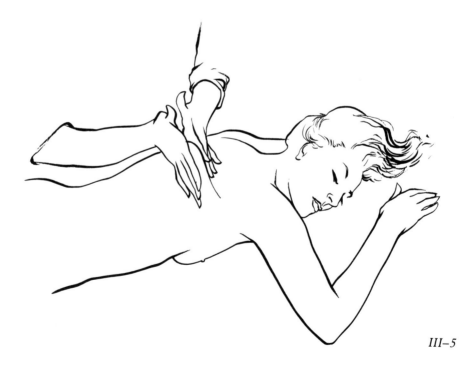

III–5

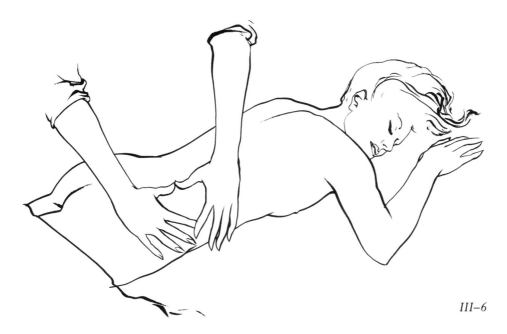

III–6

motion should be continued up the back to the shoulder, then repeated on the left side. However, because you're standing on the left side, you will find that your thumbs now move over the body and down to the table before the fingers. Rake both sides of the back, from bottom to top, three times. This movement also loosens tissue, and untangles spinal nerves.

### 10. Sweeping Oil onto the Buttocks

Pull the towel down well below the buttocks and pour another teaspoonful of oil into the palm of your hand. Sweep your hands around the buttocks, with the right hand over the left cheek and the left hand over the right cheek, four times to spread in the oil and awaken the area.

### 11. Circling the Hip

With your thumb tips together and moving in unison, make little circles from the bottom of the tailbone to about three inches above it. (See Illustration III–7.) Then bring your thumbs over the hip and down to the table or floor. Start again at the base of the tail and repeat the entire movement

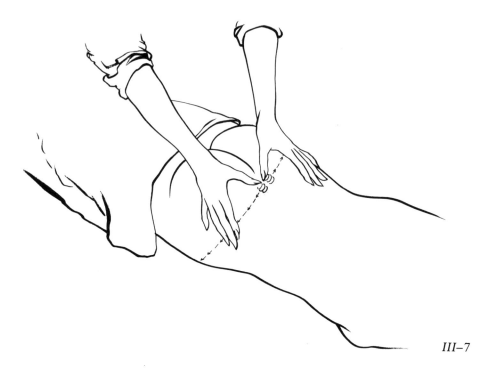

*III–7*

three times. This circling technique should be done lightly, but firmly enough so that your partner can feel it. It helps to relax the tension that contributes to lower back pain.

## 12. Running Your Thumbs on the Buttocks

This movement is wonderful for women, because it can relieve problems they have with the uterus, bladder, and sexual organs. As you work on the buttocks area, many women will tell you it feels tender; however, this technique should break up a lot of congestion, and after a few treatments the area won't feel as sore. Men, especially those with lower back or sciatic pain, will also benefit from the movement. (The pair of sciatic nerves run from deep into the buttocks down the back of each thigh.) Place your two thumbs in a parallel position at the bottom of the buttocks, about an inch out from its division on either side. Run the thumbs up through the buttock tissue to the top (some people have dimples here) and sweep them around the hip and down to the table or floor. (See Illustration III–8.) Then move your thumbs to the bottom of the buttocks again, but this time an inch closer to the outside. Repeat the movement, running up the buttock and around and down to the table again. Work in this pattern until you reach the outer sides of the buttock (or lower hip), moving out an inch at a time. Then return to the first position and repeat the sequence three more times.

### 13. Soothing the Buttock Area

After the decongesting process, the buttock now needs to be soothed. To do so, sweep your hands around the contours of each cheek, right hand on right side, left hand on left, ending with your hands flat on the center of each cheek. Hold your hands there for a moment, letting your own energy calm and revitalize the area. (The simple act of "laying on hands" can be effective therapy for any part of the body, as ancient healers well knew. The center of your hand contains a potent life force, which Eastern philosophers call a *chakra*, or opening. We make much use of this primal power during Aromatherapy massage.)

### 14. Stroking the Kidney Area

Pour a bit more oil into the palm of your hand, rub your hands together, and with the flat of both hands massage the kidney area at the small of the

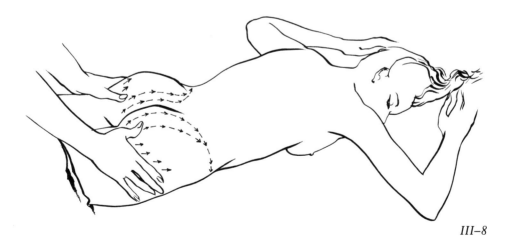

*III–8*

back with short, firm, friction strokes. Repeat about ten times. (See Illustration III–9.) This movement will help the kidneys to eliminate more efficiently—which is especially important for someone who holds water—and will stimulate the adrenals (the glands that sit on top of the kidneys and control, among other vital functions, your immune system).

### 15. Pressing the Arms and Hands

If your massage partner's arms are not lying straight out, at his side, and on the table, palms up, gently put them there. Press your thumbs into four meridian points. (See Illustration III–10.) Begin with the point in the shoulder just above the crease of the arm (see Illustration III–11); slide down and press the second point in the inner center fold at the elbow; slide down to the inner center of the wrist and press the third point just above the hand; finally, press the fourth point in the center of the hand. These are acupressure points that affect lymph circulation and metabolism (shoulder point), lung-heart function (arm), and the kidneys and adrenal glands (hand). When you finish pressing the point in the hands, give the fingers a stroking pull, and then flick your own fingers to remove any negative energy. Repeat the shoulder/arm/hand presses three times on each side.

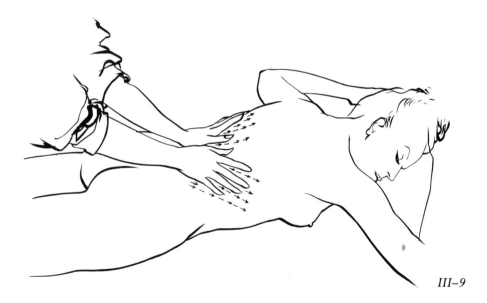

III–9

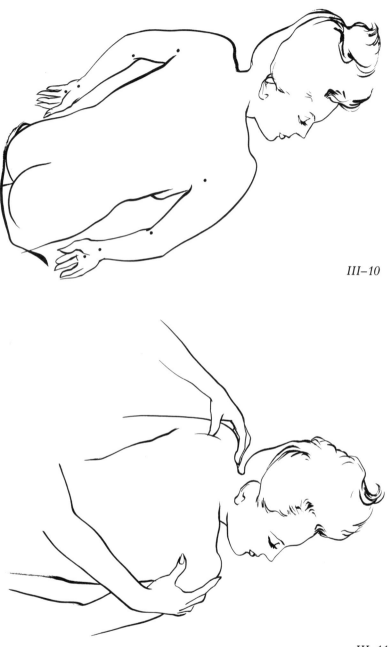

III–10

III–11

## 16. Relaxing Tension in the Neck and Shoulder Area

A tense massage partner will love you for this. Pour more oil into the palm of your hand, then firmly stroke the upper half of the back and shoulder area. Beginning with the right side, use both hands to massage around the shoulder blade and over the shoulder. With your thumb dig in and around the edge of the shoulder blade up to the neck. You may find ropey knots that are caused by tension and feel tiny crystals formed by lactic acid buildup. Work on these with your thumbs, or with the middle three fingers, making small circles and pausing with a short back-and-forth jiggling movement. The object is to break up the congestion, but *don't* dig into painful areas for more than about six seconds. The muscles and tissue get fed up with the intrusion and start to fight back. When they do they constrict, and the area can become more tense and painful than it was before. You can go back to a painful point and give it another go-round after it has had a minute or so to recover. Repeat all these movements on the left side.

Continue to massage the upper back into the neck area. Have your partner tilt his head forward so that you can work your fingers into the neck and the base of the skull. This is a very sensitive area, so take it easy, but be firm enough to smooth tense muscles and nerves. Finish the upper back area with nice upward strokes that run from mid-back up and to the outside of the shoulders. Then cover the area and keep it warm to enhance the extra circulation you have set into motion.

## 17. Preparing to Work on the Legs and Feet

You will now begin to work on the legs and feet—important movements, as they affect the entire body. Fold back the towel or sheet to the base of the buttocks. If your partner is nude, twist the bottom half of the sheet or towel and place in between his legs so that the crotch area is covered. This makes a shy person feel more secure and, depending on whom you're massaging, may make you feel more comfortable, too. Pour a teaspoonful of oil in your palm and stroke it onto one leg and foot. Repeat the process on the other side. Don't oil the feet too heavily, because they may become slippery, and you won't be able to get the necessary leverage for the deep work to follow.

Standing or kneeling at the end of the table, place your entire hand on the sole of each foot; your left hand is on the left foot, your right hand is on the right foot. (See Illustration III–12.) This is a movement borrowed from the polarity school of body work, which utilizes human magnetism to calm and stimulate. In this position you are charging the body with two poles of the same polarity (that is, right to right); because you are using a flat hand, the effect is calming and energizing. Hold your hands on your partner's feet for at least ten seconds, or even longer if you both have the time. The warmth you inspire should be gratifying for both of you.

### 18. Sliding Up the Legs

Curve your hands around your partner's anklebones for two counts. Then, run your two flat hands up to the backs of the knees. The pressure should be firm, unless the legs are spongy, which indicates they are holding water. In this case, *always* press lightly. It is not only painful to work deeply on watery tissue, but dangerous. You can harm the tissue and set too much toxic lymph flowing into the system, making your massage partner feel quite ill. People who have congested tissues are desperately in need of Aromatherapy treatment, but proceed lightly at first until the skin and shape of the leg begin to look more normal. Pause with the hands on the backs of the knees for two counts. Now continue to run your hands on up the legs with the hands flat and fingers pointing slightly to the outside of each leg. Finish by sliding your hands off the very tops of the thighs on the outside. (The lower part of the leg and back of the knee contain meridians that affect

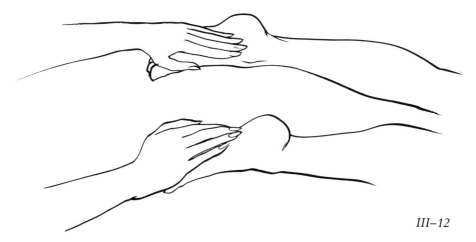

*III–12*

the thyroid, adrenals, pancreas, and gallbladder, and even this gentle sliding motion stimulates energy, sugar metabolism, and digestion.)

### 19. Foot, Ankle, and Knee Massage

You will continue to work on the feet, ankles, and knees to stimulate internal organs and liberate the lymph. Use your thumbs to make circular movements on the soles of the feet, working your way up from toes to heel. Then make the same circular movements around the ankles. You will be affecting many areas of the body with this foot massage, since the invisible channels of energy called the meridians start in the feet and run up to the top of the head. (Consult the foot chart, Diagram 9, on page 93 in Chapter 4 for a detailed map of which parts of the feet affect specific body parts and organs.) The female and male sexual organs are stimulated by ankle massage. From the ankles slide up the back of the leg to the knee again, and rest your hands there for two counts. Now slide up to just below the buttocks and with the thumbs press the lymphatic points that are nestled at the base, about three inches out from the division on each side. (See Illustration III–13.) This is

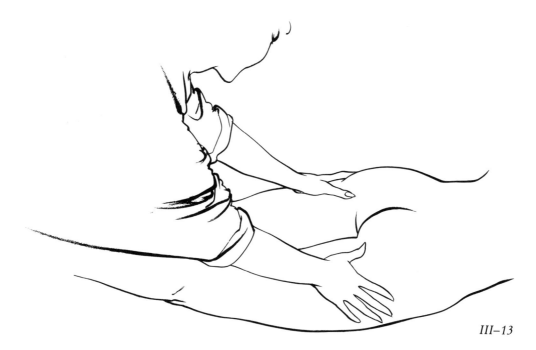

III–13

a tricky movement, but worth perfecting; you and your partner will instinctively know when you have the right points under your thumbs. This is an excellent technique for stimulating lymph flow.

Repeat Movements 18 and 19 three times each, resting the hands on the soles of the feet for ten seconds at the end.

You are now ready to begin work on the head, neck, and chest. Pick up the towel or sheet and ask your partner to turn over. Replace the towel or sheet, leaving the neck and shoulders uncovered, then wash your hands, which have been working on the feet, before you touch the face.

### 20. Pressing the Head with Your Thumbs

Sit on a stool at your massage partner's head and, with dry hands, begin pressing the forehead with your thumbs. Put one thumb on top of the other to enhance the pressure, and press at one-inch intervals, starting from the center of the top of the forehead, then moving over the top of the head to the back of the head, and down toward the neck as far as you can go. (See Illustration III–14.) This movement affects a very important "governing" meridian that reaches down to the anus, and stimulates the master pituitary gland, which communicates to other glands. Repeat three times.

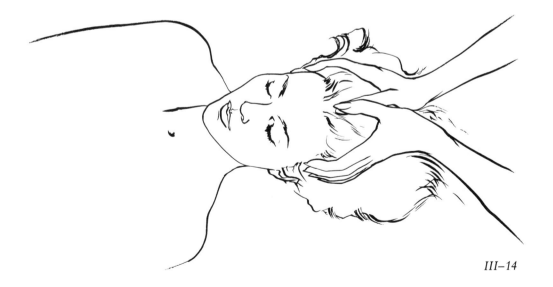

III–14

## 21. Stimulating the Scalp

With your fingers spread, firmly massage the scalp all over. Hold your fingers in one place at a time and actually *move* the scalp. (Don't let your fingers slide around on the hair.) This loosens the scalp, bringing a nourishing flow of blood to the hair follicles, and stimulates nerve endings that relieve tension in the head.

## 22. Magnetic Cleansing

Rake your fingers through the hair, starting at the scalp. Pull through to the very tips of the hair, giving your hands a flick as you reach the ends. This "cleansing" action draws out negative magnetic charges from the head and the hair. Repeat six times.

## 23. Applying Oil to the Face and Upper Body

Pour half a teaspoonful of face oil into the palm of one hand, rub your hands together, and apply it to the face, working both hands in unison on each side of the face, over the nose and chin, and carefully around the eyes. Work evenly, and take care not to get oil in your partner's eyes. Put a bit more oil in your hands and stroke it upward around the neck, then out over the chest and shoulders. You can use the same oil for both the body and face, but I prefer a lighter blend for the face. If you haven't mixed a special face oil yet, you can dilute the body oil with a little safflower, sunflower, or sesame oil.

## 24. Pressing the Forehead

With your two thumbs facing each other, start just above the eyebrows in the center of the forehead and press in a straight line out to the hairline on the side of the head; press in at one-inch intervals. Repeat the movement, this time pressing in at half-inch intervals and moving up, until you reach the hairline at the forehead. (See Illustration III–15.) Return to the area above the brows and repeat both series of presses three times. This stimulates digestion and elimination. Remember that the facial area is small and sensitive; be definite with your movements, but never rough. You should use the same light, flexible touch you use to touch your own face.

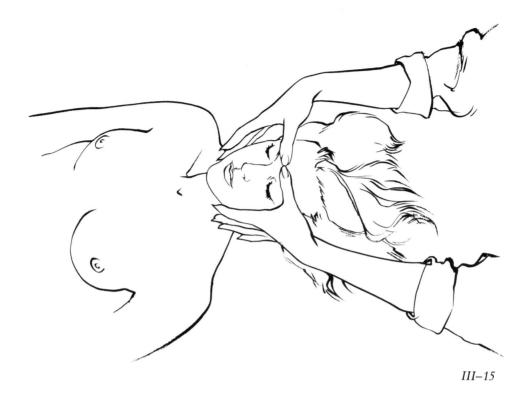

*III–15*

### 25. Brushing the Forehead

Place your hands horizontally on your partner's forehead, one hand several inches above the other. With a rolling motion (as if you were brushing crumbs off a table), brush one hand over the forehead, the other hand following. The center of your palm is most in contact with the head, and the pinky comes off last, as you roll your hand. (See Illustration III–16.) This soothing, hypnotic movement can be done between all movements on the top of the face.

### 26. Pressing the Bridge of the Nose

Press your thumbs, using the right and left thumbs alternately, into the bridge of the nose, using short, upward-sliding motions. This movement relieves the sinuses, and stimulates the liver and stomach meridians.

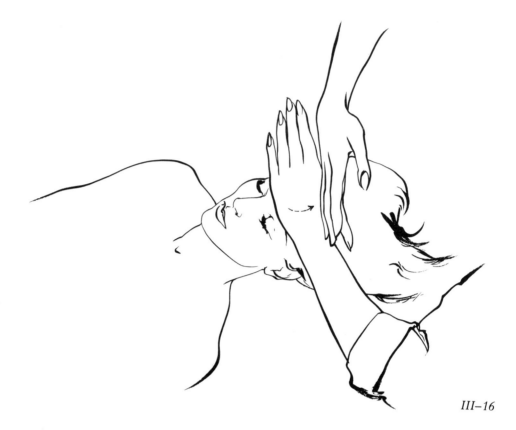

*III–16*

### 27. Circling the Eyes

With either your second or middle fingers, circle the eyes, starting from the inside corner of the eyebrows and moving out and around below the eyes. (See Illustration III–17.) Every second circle cross over the eyelid and come up toward the brow. Exert more pressure over the brow, and very light pressure over the eyelid. Repeat six times. This movement calms and revives the eye and stimulates the meridian that affects the liver and digestion.

### 28. Pinching the Eyebrows

Firmly pinch the bone above the eyes (just under the brows) beginning on the inside near the nose and working outward with small movements until you reach the end of the brow. Repeat three times. This is good for the eyes and sinuses and stimulates the digestion meridian.

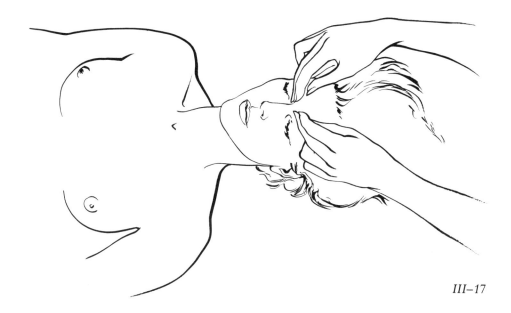

*III–17*

### 29. Decongesting the Nose

With the third fingers of both hands make little circles on each side of the base of the nose, working up to the bridge. Then slide your fingers over the forehead to the hairline. Be sure that you don't prevent your partner from breathing for more than a second, which you can do if you pinch the nostrils or press too hard on the sides of the nose. Repeat three times. This decongests the nose and stimulates the lung meridian—an excellent technique for a partner who is coming down with a cold. If the sinuses are stuffed up, or if your partner has a cough, put a pillow under the head when your partner is lying face up. This will keep fluid from blocking the breathing passages.

### 30. Raking the Cheeks

Spread four fingers of each hand over the cheeks on each side of the nose. With firm pressure "rake" over the cheek to the ear. Repeat six times. (See Illustration III–18.) This helps drain the sinuses and benefits the lymph capillaries that run horizontally across the face into the lymph glands in the jawbone under the ear.

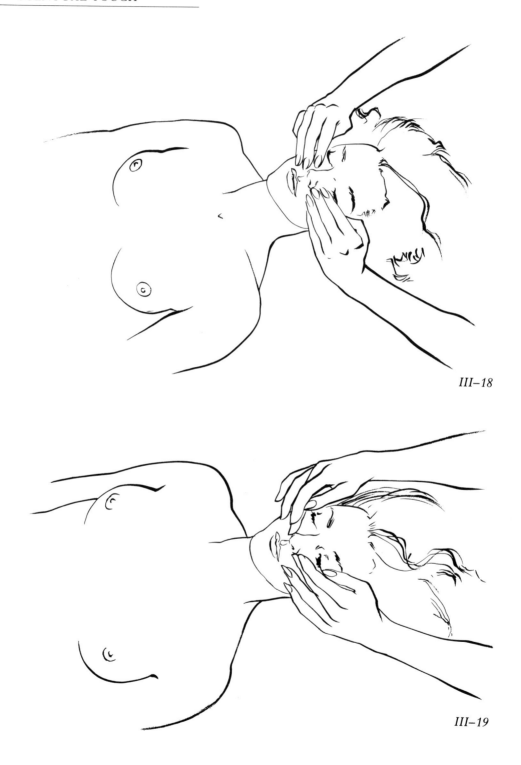

III–18

III–19

### 31. Stimulating the "Chinese Point"

Just under the cheekbone at the nostrils is an area with the romantic name "Chinese point." Perhaps it was essential to some ancient Chinese cure; in any case, the Chinese point is a lung point, and pressure on this point does relieve congested sinuses, and affects the large intestine. Press at the nostrils with the first two fingers of each hand, holding for a count of ten, then finish by sweeping four fingers of each hand out to the ear. (See Illustration III–19.) Repeat both the press and the sweep three times.

### 32. Liberating the Lymph in the Lower Face

Spread the four fingers of each hand, placing two fingers over the upper lip and two on the chin; then "rake" outward to the ears. This encourages the lymph to flow into the nodes at the sides of the lower jaw, called mandibular lymph nodes. (See Diagram 6.)

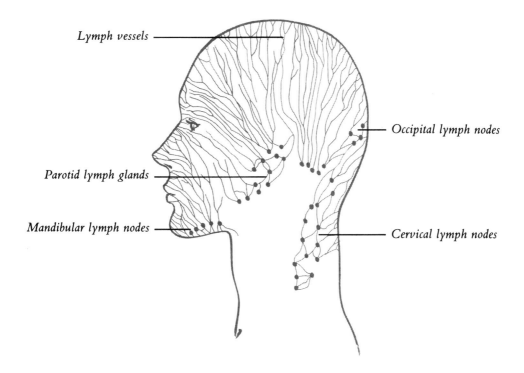

**HEAD LYMPH NODES AND VESSELS**
*Diagram 6*

### 33. Stimulating the Chin/Jaw Area

Place your fingers under your partner's jaw and, beginning at the center, make little circles with your thumbs outward to the ears. (See Illustration III–20.) This tones the chin line and affects the meridian that governs the stomach and small intestines. Repeat three times.

### 34. Toning the Neck

Holding your left hand under the neck, slide your right hand around the front of the neck, working from left to right. Now change hands, placing the right hand underneath the neck, and sliding with the left. (See Illustration III–21.) You should use a flat hand and make sure the neck is sufficiently oiled so that you won't pull the skin. This tones the skin on the neck and prepares it for the next movement. Repeat left and right three times each.

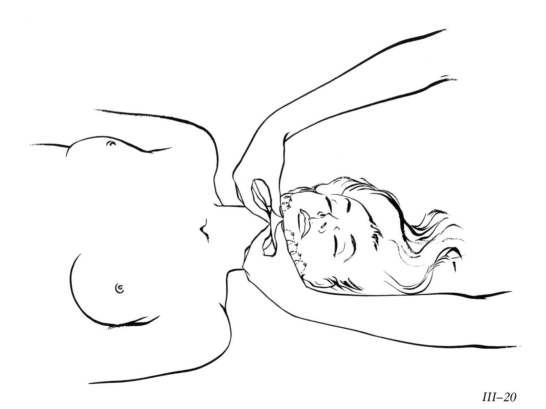

III–20

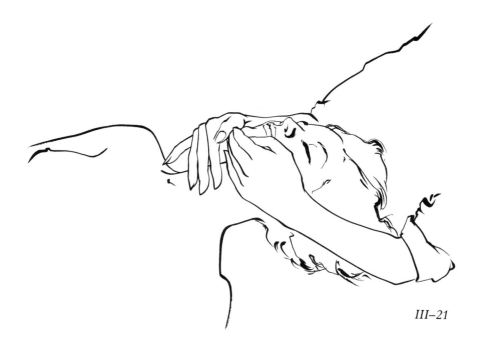

*III–21*

### 35. Stimulating Lymph and Nerve Points from Neck to Chest

This is a large movement that touches on many important points. Begin by sliding your hands from the base of the neck over the collarbone down to the area just above the breast; hold your hands about four inches apart. Pause here and press for two counts. (See Illustration III–22.) Then sweep your hands over to the top of the shoulders and press them down, holding for two counts. Finally run your hands all the way up the sides of the neck and head and out through the hair. (This movement and some of the other movements will make the hair a little oily, but it is worth it to experience the complete movement. If your partner objects to oil in the hair, you can discontinue certain movements at the hairline once your hands have become oily.) Repeat the entire process three times. As you move down the chest you are passing over lymph nodes and the large lymph vessels and nerve points that affect the thyroid, kidneys, and lungs. The press above the breast affects the liver and gallbladder, and the shoulder press is thought to relieve brain fatigue. Quite a list for one movement!

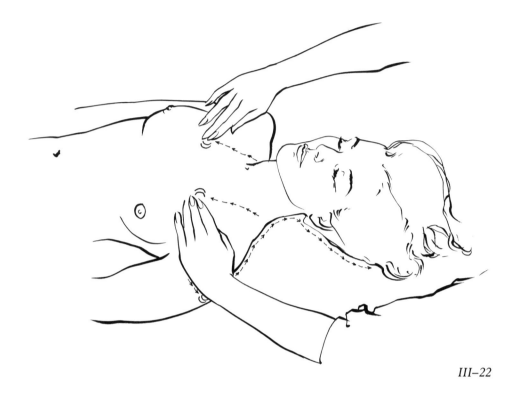

*III–22*

### 36. Massaging the Back of the Shoulder

Slip your hands under your partner's shoulders, close to the spine. With a circular motion, massage the shoulder blades, upper back, and shoulders. (See Illustration III–23.) Rest your lower arms on the table for more leverage. This is more difficult to do if you are kneeling on the floor. This movement is excellent for relieving upper back tension.

### 37. Massaging the Front and Back of the Shoulders

Still moving your fingers in circles, work firmly around the top, front, and sides of the shoulders. If your partner is a woman, pay special attention to the bone at the base of the neck, which often grows an unattractive "hump" in middle age. Massaging this hump can help break up the fat and calcium deposits that form it.

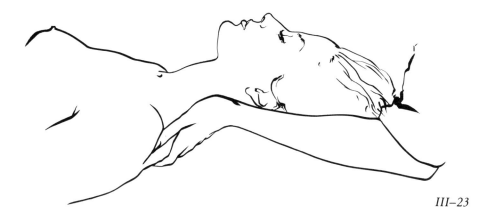

*III–23*

### 38. Stimulating the Lymph Point in the Collarbone
Sliding from the neck down to the midpoints under the collarbones, press with your first two fingers for a count of two, using both hands. (See Illustration III–24.) Then with circling movements work your way out to the end of the shoulders and slide up the sides of the neck and head and off through the hair. You are stimulating lung points as well as liberating the lymph.

### 39. Calming and Reviving the Diaphragm
Roll down the sheet or blanket covering your partner to the top of the thighs. If you are massaging a woman and she is shy, you can put a small towel over her breasts. Pour a scant teaspoonful of oil in your hand and sweep it over the stomach and diaphragm (which covers the area from under the breast to the waist). Make sure you don't get this area too oily, because your hands will slip and slide and have less control. Now put your left hand on your partner's right arm, and your right hand on the center of the diaphragm, your fingers pointing up toward the breast. Gently jiggle the right hand to send a friendly, restorative message to your partner's nervous system. (See Illustration III–25.) Keeping your left hand on your partner's arm, inscribe a counterclockwise circle with the flat of your hand all around the

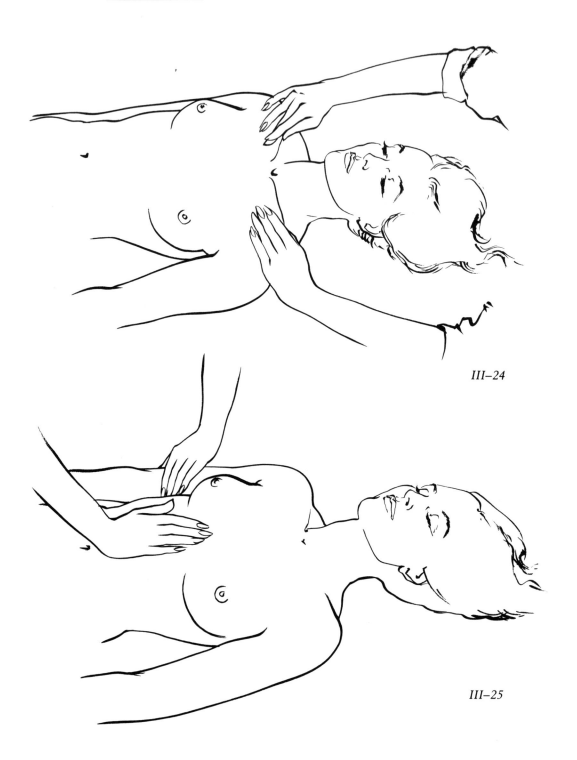

III—24

III—25

diaphragm area. Make this circle six times, moving slowly, and concentrating on putting your most healing energy into the movement. The diaphragm is a key nerve and lymph center, containing deep lymphatic vessels and cranial nerves that carry impulses from the organs to the brain. To calm a nervous partner, hold a warm, caring hand on the diaphragm.

### 40. Massaging the Feet

A foot massage is a wonderful if slightly weird experience. Before beginning, cover your partner's body and chest and roll back the other end of the sheet to expose the legs. You may want to twist the towel or sheet between the legs again. Pour about a teaspoonful of oil into your palm and sweep it up one leg with both hands. Do the same to the other leg. Once again, pour a small amount of oil into your palm; then rub it into the feet. With the wrists tilted inward, grasp the tops of the feet with your fingers, the thumbs on the heels. Now slide up the feet with your thumbs from the heel to the big toe. Do this three times starting at the inner side of the foot and working toward the center. (See Illustration III–26.) When you can't go any farther in this position, move the hands to the outside of the feet and, grasping the tops of the feet with the fingers, work the thumbs up from the heel to the

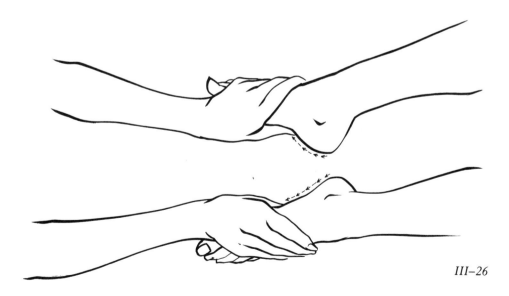

III–26

big toe. Do this three times working from the outside of the foot toward the center. (See Illustration III–27.) This is a strong movement and should be done with gusto in order to stimulate the entire system.

### 41. Liberating the Lymph in the Feet

Hold the soles of the feet with your fingers. At the same time, stroke between the toes in the direction of the ankle with your thumbs. This encourages the lymph that flows down to the toes to start its upward journey to the nodes in the knees. Besides, it feels good. Work the feet, moving from big toes to little toes, several times.

### 42. Stimulating Ankles, Knees, and Legs

Sliding your hands from the feet to the ankles, massage them with a circular motion. This is beneficial for female organs. Then slide your flat hands up to the knees and rest them there for two counts. The popliteal lymph nodes that drain the bottom of the legs are located in the front of the knees, so by sliding up the leg and resting your warm hands on the knees you are en-

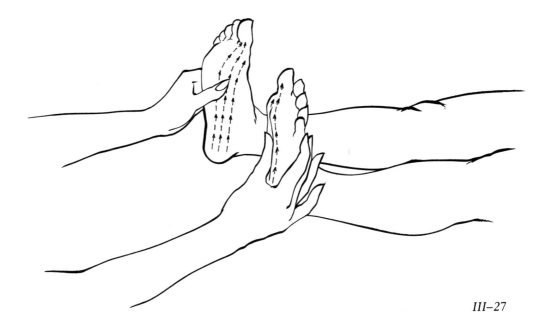

III–27

couraging the lymph to travel into these nodes, where it is processed. From the knees slide up to the groin and press in with your thumbs to stimulate the inguinal lymph nodes there. (See Illustration III–28.) These nodes are located about two inches in from the center thigh at its very top. This cleansing, stimulating movement should be done gently; it usually makes people jump because the area is sensitive. Repeat these movements three times.

### 43. Ending the Treatment

End your Aromatherapy treatment by placing the flats of your hands on the soles of your massage partner's feet, with your right hand on the left foot and your left hand on the right foot. Now you are creating a positive-negative charge in the body, which is calming, stops muscle contraction, and wakes up the nervous system. Hold this position for a count of twenty then slowly withdraw your hands and cover the legs with the sheet or towel. Let your partner relax for a few moments and relish the ethereal, floating sensation and delicious fragrance. If your partner falls sound asleep (which often happens), awaken gently in order not to disrupt the deep calm that is restoring vitality and a feeling of well-being.

Remember to wash your hands when you've finished the treatment and give them a good shake to release any negative magnetism.

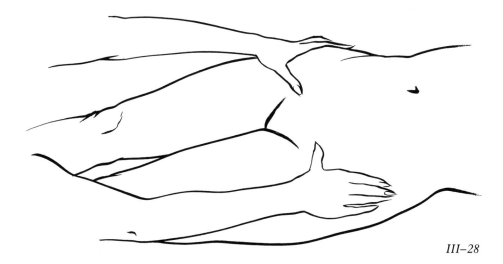

III–28

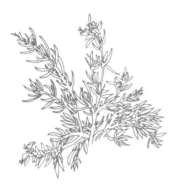

## IV

# SCENTUAL SELF-MASSAGE

Most of us lack a physical sense of self and know little about how the complex human machine that houses our intellect and emotions actually functions. In the psychology-oriented twentieth century, when we think of our "selves" we tend to think about our minds, and even blame our psyches for physical problems. We relegate our body awareness to critical or admiring glances in the bathroom mirror and to what our doctors are willing to confide about our cholesterol levels and blood pressure counts. Few of us devote much time or energy to exploring our own bodies with our eyes, let alone our fingers. Have you ever experienced the shape or texture of your limbs and torso? Do you know what your elbow feels like, or if the backs of your legs are smooth or lumpy? Even those figure-conscious people, interested in the way their bodies look, tend to restrict their view to the top and front sides, and the vast majority of the three trillion cells that comprise their corpus delecti remain virtual strangers.

We owe some of our limited body sense to Victorian taboos. In the nineteenth century, formal social relations prohibited intimate touch, and nudity was for statues, whose idealized forms and camouflaged private parts represented aesthetics from the Grecian era. Victorian fashions made the body almost invisible, much less touchable. A mere century later, the pendulum has swung to the opposite extreme—to skin flicks, nude beaches, revealing fashions, and the recent fitness craze. Most of us, however, are stranded somewhere between the nineteenth century and modern times— we no longer deny our bodies, yet we are not completely comfortable with them either.

Aromatherapy self-massage will teach you about your inner body by literally putting you in touch with its outer covering. Through this exciting process of self-discovery, you will learn there is more to your body than your mirror reveals. Self-touch will allow you to take more control over how your body feels and functions. It can enable you to treat minor health problems without drugs, and because it gives you a clear, tactile picture of your body, it can make you more aware of changes when they do occur, including early symptoms of potentially serious diseases. Self-massage will also make you more sensuously aware; it will show you what kind of touch you find stimulating, calming, or erotic. You will learn which parts of yourself are sensitive, tense, or even easily aroused. (With luck, you may discover personal, uncharted erogenous zones.) Moreover, by touching yourself you will discover the secrets of touching others effectively. (Some of the movements in self-massage are the same as, or similar to, those you used in the basic massage.) You will learn what intensity of movement is most effective, and how muscles, nerves, and internal organs respond to the different techniques. Acquiring a personalized self-touch system can also give you access to some of the important health benefits of exercise. When time, space, recent illness, or injury prohibits athletic huffing and puffing, Aromatherapy can substitute, stimulating the nerves, glands, and circulation. Finally, Aromatherapy self-massage will enable you to treat yourself to the relaxing and enjoyable combination of the deliciously fragrant nourishing oils and therapeutic touch. You will be able to use these techniques to increase your energy to decrease tension, to relieve minor aches and pains. These touch techniques can be done anywhere—in the home, office, hotel, or jet—without anyone else, or any special equipment.

## ___ SELF-TOUCH TECHNIQUE___

Aromatherapy self-massage is easy, and *almost* as effective as a full-scale treatment on a massage therapist's table. I say "almost" because there are places that are tricky to reach with your own hands—like the upper middle of your back—and because another person's skillful touch and magnetic energy can give your body an extra charge.

The techniques you will use for your self-massage are similar to those you mastered in the last chapter. They are also based on an Eastern system of self-massage called "Dō-In," which is a combination of Oriental treatment techniques. Like acupuncture and Shiatsu, Dō-In is based on the idea that by pressing specific points we unblock energy in the meridian channels, which run, like connective highways, through various parts of the body. As you read my directions for relieving eyestrain, headache, and other problems, you may be surprised to discover that these vital points are far from the area that seems to be adversely affected; pressing them, however, will unblock energy "traffic jams" down the entire meridian and relieve the troublesome congestion. In my instructions, I will tell you where the important points are located, and you can also consult the meridian chart (Diagram 7). You will be pressing these points and manipulating parts of your body with the following touch techniques:

| | |
|---|---|
| Stroking | Pressing |
| Grasping | Pulling |
| Tapping | Pounding |
| Kneading | Pinching |

You will also be "laying on hands" on yourself, a self-polarity technique, in which you will be using your own hands to transfer stimulating and calming charges from one part of your body to another. "Self-polarity" is especially effective to ease headache pain and tension.

## ___ THE WAKE-UP MASSAGE ___

The series of movements that follows can send you into your day feeling well-balanced and energized. But before you begin the massage, you should prepare yourself with some scented stretching and breathing preliminaries.

· Although the self-touch wake-up is done with dry hands, fragrance can enhance its effects. Warm a few drops of essential oil in your heater, or on a light bulb to scent the room. Rub just a drop of neat (undiluted) essential oil into your hands; use juniper for energy, lavender for calming,

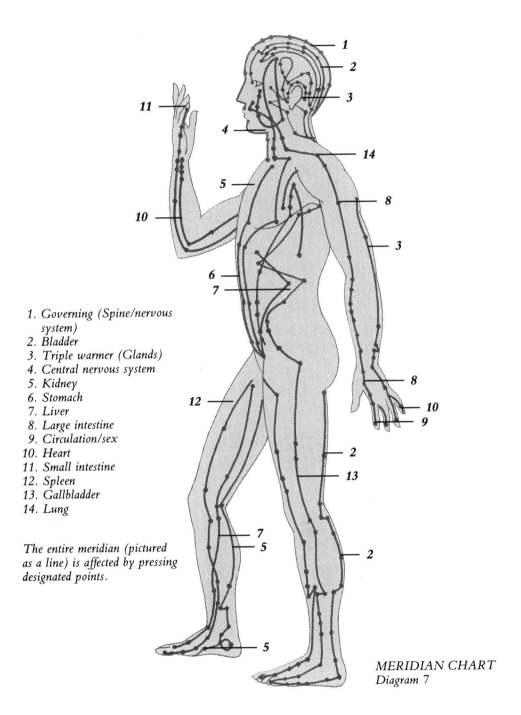

1. Governing (Spine/nervous system)
2. Bladder
3. Triple warmer (Glands)
4. Central nervous system
5. Kidney
6. Stomach
7. Liver
8. Large intestine
9. Circulation/sex
10. Heart
11. Small intestine
12. Spleen
13. Gallbladder
14. Lung

*The entire meridian (pictured as a line) is affected by pressing designated points.*

MERIDIAN CHART
*Diagram 7*

· eucalyptus or pine for decongesting. Try incense if you feel slightly head-achey or toxic and hung over. Peppermint cools and refreshes on a hot morning; patchouli warms and braces you for a cold one.

· Lie on the floor and relax totally, breathing deeply from the stomach, bringing the air down into your diaphragm, then on up to fill the chest; exhale fully through the nose. After about six breaths, bring one knee up to the chest and hold it there with your arms around it for a count of six. Repeat with the other leg. Stretch both legs three times, then bring both knees to the chest and hold for a count of six, three times. (See Illustration IV–1.) This simple exercise should stretch your lower back and legs so that the series can be done more comfortably.

Begin the movements by sitting on your heels with your back straight; you should be on the floor, but if it is too hard for your anatomy, sit up straight on the edge of a chair. Take a deep breath, bringing life-affirming oxygen down into your diaphragm, and then exhale deeply. Make sure you breathe deeply and naturally while you are doing the movements. Take a deep breath between each move and consciously relax. Concentrate on what

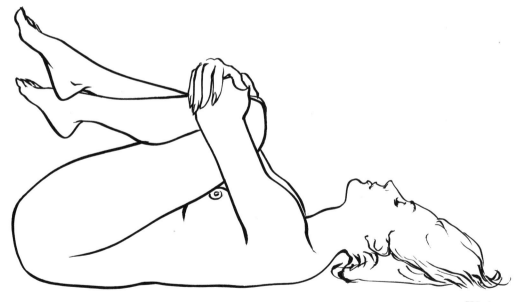

IV–1

you are doing, as you want to wake up your brain as well as your body. Now begin.

### 1. Yin-Yang Clap

Rub both hands together briskly and then clap them sharply twice. According to Oriental philosophy, this clap brings opposing forces of the body, the yin and the yang, together. It does seem to start off the rest of the movements with a bang!

### 2. Shoulder-Arm Tap

Hold your left arm above the elbow with your right hand. Cross the left arm over, and forcefully tap your right shoulder area with your left fist. Let go of your left arm and continue tapping down the inside of the right arm and up the outside. Tap hard, moving down and up three times. Repeat. Then move to the left side, holding the right arm with the left hand to begin tapping the left shoulder. This movement relieves tension in the neck and shoulder area, and stimulates the lungs, heart, circulation, sexual organs, and intestines.

### 3. Head-Face Tap

Shake your hands to remove any negative vibrations and tap the top of your head with the tips of your fingers, making a large counterclockwise circle with both hands moving in one direction. Tap across the forehead and down the face. End by slapping your jawline. (See Illustration IV–2.) Repeat several times. This gets the circulation going all over your head and face. I feel that it wakes up my brains.

### 4. Head Pressures

With your fingertips placed at the top of the forehead, press them over the head, all the way down to the back of the neck. The fingers of both hands should be lined up about an inch apart; both hands should work in unison over the head. Repeat six times. (See Illustration IV–3.) This movement is stimulating to the cranial nerves and to the master of the glands, the pituitary.

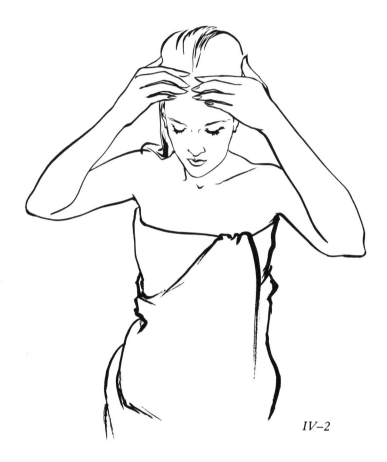

*IV–2*

### 5. Eyebrow Pinch

Squeeze along your eyebrows with your thumb and index finger. Begin at the nose and squeeze the entire length of the brow. Repeat three times. This helps wake up tired eyes and unblocks sinuses. The meridian in the eyebrow also affects digestion.

### 6. Chinese Point Sinus Slide

The Chinese point is a lung point located at the nostrils. To stimulate the lungs and decongest the sinuses, press in at the side of each nostril for two counts with your middle fingers, then slide your fingers under the cheekbone out to the ear. Repeat three times.

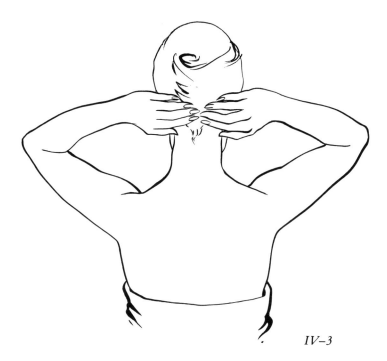

*IV–3*

### 7. Ear Flaps and Pressures

Put your hands behind your ears and brush them forward with small, flapping motions. Then press around the ridge of the outer ear, working toward the ridges on the inside. The ear is an important part of the body from the Oriental healer's point of view. Its shape relates it to early fetal development and the kidneys. (See Diagram 8.) The entire ear contains points that relate to organs, glands, nerves, circulation, digestion and elimination, and body parts. Study the ear chart (Diagram 8) and experiment with pressure, noting the results. The ear is a convenient therapy tool, since you can reach it easily and press it anywhere. Try this movement the next time you are stuck in a boring movie, or on a long airplane flight.

### 8. Base-of-the-Skull Pressures

Rest your thumbs at the base of the skull and slide your hands up under your hair on each side of your head. Then press firmly with the thumbs

1. Fingers
2. Thumb
3. Toes
4. Ankle
5. Knee joint
6. Allergies
7. Sciatic nerve
8. Pubic region
9. Ovaries and testes
10. Bladder
11. Large intestine
12. Small intestine
13. Bronchial tubes
14. Stomach and digestion
15. Lung
16. Adrenal gland
17. Neck, throat, thyroid
18. Senses
19. Sexual organs
20. Thalamus
21. Dizziness
22. Upper digestive tract
23. Rejuvenation point
24. Heart
25. Spleen
26. Gallbladder
27. Liver
28. Kidney
29. Coccyx
30. Wrists
31. Elbows
32. Chest
33. Clavicle and sternum
34. Shoulder joint

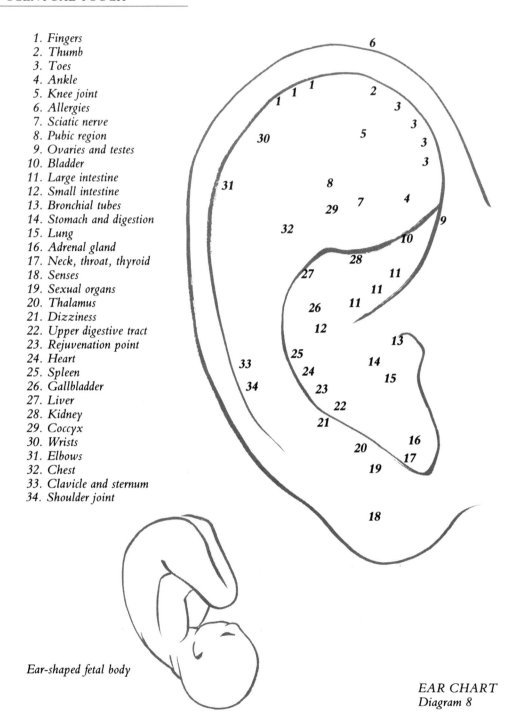

Ear-shaped fetal body

EAR CHART
Diagram 8

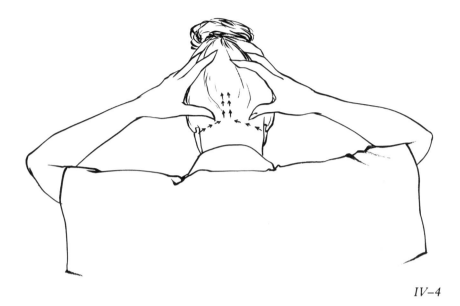

*IV–4*

all along the base of the skull, and up into the middle of the head. Repeat three times. (See Illustration IV–4.) You are stimulating the nerves that cross from the spine to the brain and lymph glands, and reawakening the entire body.

### 9. Neck Pressures

Place your fingers on each side of the neck bone (the cervical spine) and with firm pressures start at the base of the skull and work down as far as you can go until you reach the shoulder. Repeat three times. This stimulates circulation, loosens stiffness in the area, and relieves tension.

### 10. Shoulder Pinch

Grasp the flesh between your neck and shoulder on the right side with your right hand and on the left side with your left hand. Hold for two counts. Then grasp the flesh closer to the shoulder. Repeat until you reach the outside of the shoulder. (See Illustration IV–5.) This dissolves tension, which tends to accumulate in the neck and shoulders.

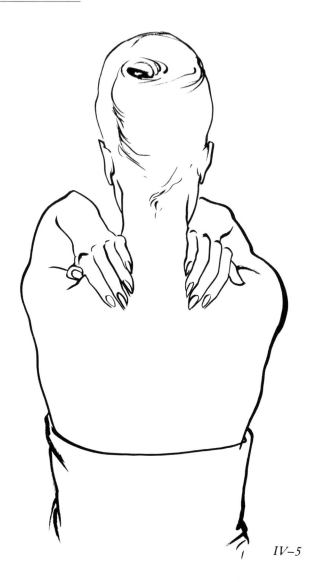

IV–5

### 11. Solar Plexus Waist Tap

With both fists pound the solar plexus (the midsection of your body between the breastbone and the waist) and the waist for ten seconds. This movement stimulates the nerve that communicates to the brain and increases the flow of blood to your vital organs.

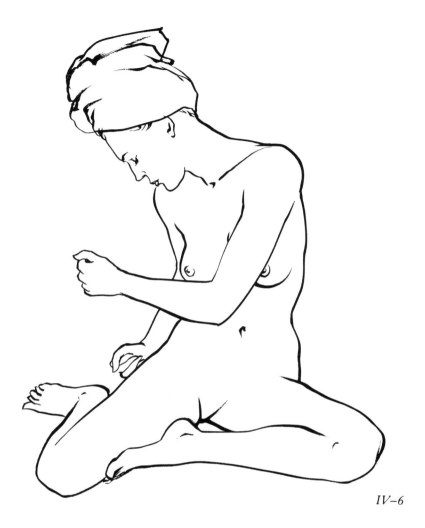

IV–6

### 12. Leg Tapping and Pressures

Sit on your left hip with your right buttock off the floor and your legs to
one side. With your fists tap down the outside and up the inside of the right
leg. (See Illustration IV–6.) Then press the inside of the lower leg bone from
ankle to knee with your thumbs. (See Illustration IV–7.) Repeat the same
movement on the left side, sitting on the right hip, with the left buttock off
the floor.

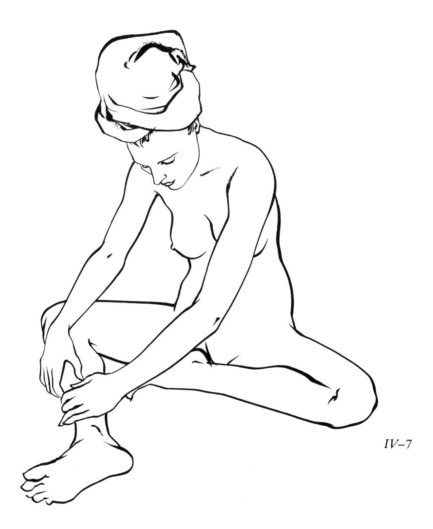

*IV–7*

### 13. Foot Pressures

Stretch out your left leg, and pull the right leg toward you, so that your knee is bent, and you can reach your foot. Pound the sole of your foot with your fist, from toe to heel. This loosens up the foot tissue and wakes up the nerves. Then, starting at the toes, press all the points noted on the foot chart (Diagram 9). Press as hard as you can with your thumb, and even with your knuckles if your skin is calloused. Then start at the top of the

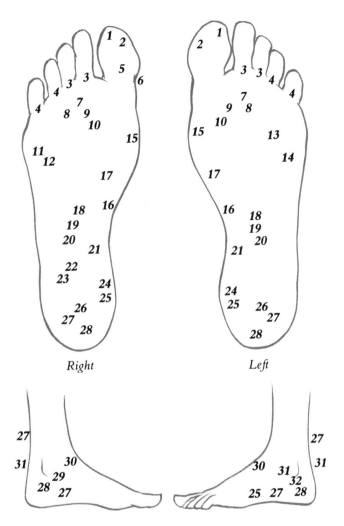

Right                    Left

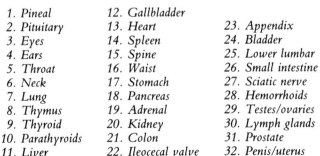

| | | |
|---|---|---|
| 1. Pineal | 12. Gallbladder | |
| 2. Pituitary | 13. Heart | 23. Appendix |
| 3. Eyes | 14. Spleen | 24. Bladder |
| 4. Ears | 15. Spine | 25. Lower lumbar |
| 5. Throat | 16. Waist | 26. Small intestine |
| 6. Neck | 17. Stomach | 27. Sciatic nerve |
| 7. Lung | 18. Pancreas | 28. Hemorrhoids |
| 8. Thymus | 19. Adrenal | 29. Testes/ovaries |
| 9. Thyroid | 20. Kidney | 30. Lymph glands |
| 10. Parathyroids | 21. Colon | 31. Prostate |
| 11. Liver | 22. Ileocecal valve | 32. Penis/uterus |

FOOT CHART
Diagram 9

foot, raking between the toes with your thumb; pull the thumb toward the ankle. This stimulates lymph flow. Then press and massage the top of the foot (especially good for women, since this is where the breast point is located) and down around the ankle, which affects the sexual organs. If you find a particular area painful, give it some extra pressure and apply the pressure for a longer time. Consult the foot chart to see which area of the body is related to the sore point. The foot can often tell you when you have a problem before other symptoms appear.

### 14. Back Stimulation

Rise up on your knees, buttocks off the feet, bend a bit forward, and pound your back with your fists. Start as high as you can reach, and work your way down to the buttocks. This awakens nerve centers and is especially good for the kidneys and adrenals, which are located in the middle of your back above the waist.

### 15. Fetal Crouch

To complete the wake-up series, relax totally in the fetal position. Sit on your knees, and bend forward with the top of your head on the ground, arms down at your sides. Feel your rejuvenated cells working to energize and support you for the rest of the day.

## ____ SELF-TOUCH FOR SPECIAL PROBLEMS____

The following techniques are effective physical and mental remedies for pain and tension. They will work even better if a drop of the right essential oil is rubbed into the hands before you begin.

### HEADACHE

A headache is a minor but crippling ailment that can be caused by eyestrain, blocked sinuses, tension, liver, stomach, or intestinal problems, and even tight shoes. The first challenge to your self-massage technique will be to see if you can discover the source of the pain. Your hands and feet and your head itself all have points that will tell you what is causing the headache; when these parts are pressed and manipulated you can bring yourself relief. The following touches usually relieve the pain, but if they should reap no results, consult the hand chart shown here (Diagram 10) and the foot chart

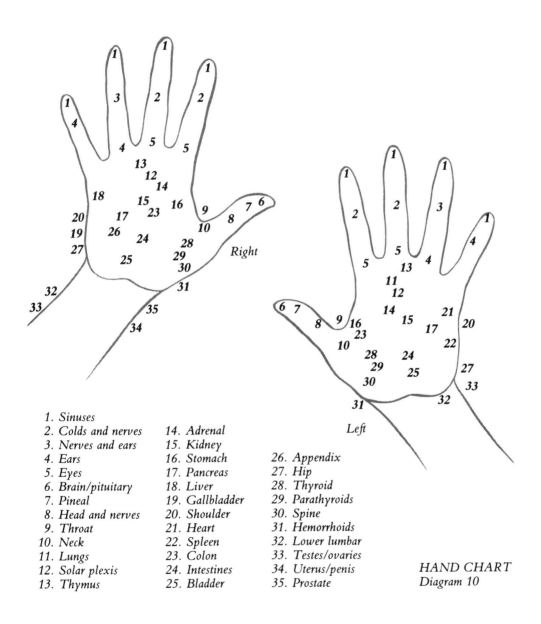

1. Sinuses
2. Colds and nerves
3. Nerves and ears
4. Ears
5. Eyes
6. Brain/pituitary
7. Pineal
8. Head and nerves
9. Throat
10. Neck
11. Lungs
12. Solar plexis
13. Thymus
14. Adrenal
15. Kidney
16. Stomach
17. Pancreas
18. Liver
19. Gallbladder
20. Shoulder
21. Heart
22. Spleen
23. Colon
24. Intestines
25. Bladder
26. Appendix
27. Hip
28. Thyroid
29. Parathyroids
30. Spine
31. Hemorrhoids
32. Lower lumbar
33. Testes/ovaries
34. Uterus/penis
35. Prostate

HAND CHART
Diagram 10

(Diagram 9) on page 93 to decide what other points you want to try. Press any of the points for a count of ten and release, pause for a moment, then try two more cycles of pressing, counting, and releasing. You will know when you find the right point because the headache pain will immediately fade. If one point doesn't work, keep trying.

### 1. Head Pressures

Place your elbows on a table or desk and with your third right finger press in at the top center of the forehead. Reinforce the pressure by pushing with the finger of your left hand over the finger of the right. (See Illustration IV–8.) Now try the double finger press two inches on either side of the center spot. These are Dō-In "governor nerve centers," and will often erase headache pain.

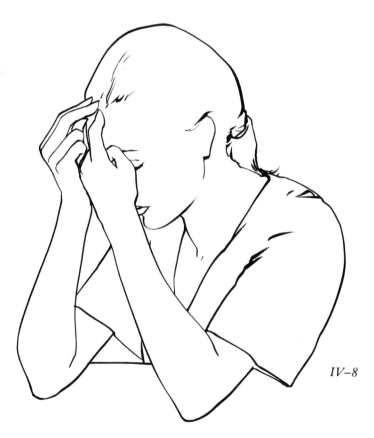

IV–8

### 2. Hand Pressures

To cause your brain to release endorphins, nature's own pain killer, squeeze the web between the index finger and the thumb of the left hand with the thumb and index finger of the right. Then press in at the side of the web, near the base of the second finger.

### 3. Finger Pinches

Pinch the ends of the middle three fingers of each hand. These are head and sinus points.

### 4. Foot Pressures and Pinches

The meridian in the big toe relates to the head and the neck. If your headache is caused by tension, it can often be relieved by grasping the big toe and circling it around and around. This should miraculously loosen up your neck. Then pinch the ends of your toes, which are sinus points.

### EYESTRAIN

When you read, or do any kind of concentrated work that keeps your eyes in the same focus for hours, it is easy to strain them. Nearsightedness, as well as discomfort, can result from "frozen focus," so it is important to learn to relax and release the muscles and nerves of the eyes. Here are some suggestions:

### 1. Face Pressures and Massage

Press with the first two fingers underneath the eyes, starting at the inner corners and working to the outer corners. These are reflex points for the kidneys and adrenal glands as well as the eyes. Do a series of six pressures. Then press the bone underneath the eyebrows with all four fingers. (See Illustration IV–9.) Hold for ten seconds. Repeat three times. Support your elbows on a table or desk to get better leverage.

### 2. Back-of-the-Head Pressures

Press the base of the skull with your thumbs, moving up into the division of the skull. Keep your hands on the side of the head while you press. Then

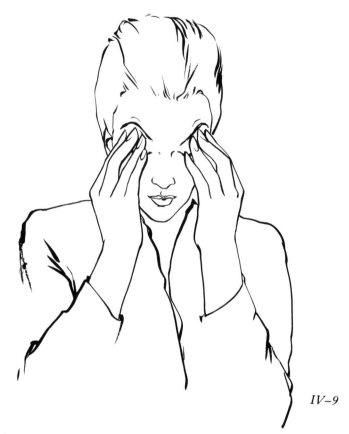

IV–9

move down the neck, pressing along the neck bone (cervical spine) with the fingers. The nerves in this area all affect the eyesight. Repeat the entire movement three times.

### 3. Palming

Place both palms over the eyes to create total darkness, but do not press in on the eyes. Hold this position for at least a minute. The warmth of your hands and the darkness relieve tension and revive circulation. Keep your elbows on a table or desk. If you are working a great deal with your eyes, try palming every hour.

### 4. Eyebrow Massage

Massage across the forehead just above the eyebrows. Starting at the center, and working with the first two fingers, press and circle out to the hairline on each side. If this area feels tight, you will know that energy to the eyes is being restricted. Now pinch the top of the nose bone that is between the eyes. Repeat six times.

### 5. Thumb Massage

The thumb, like the big toe, is related to the head and the neck. Give each thumb a good massage, pressing and kneading, to relieve tension in the entire head area, including the eyes.

### 6. Toe Presses

The eye reflexes are located at the bottom of the second and third toes, close to the foot. Hold your foot up so that you can work efficiently on this area. With your thumb press and then rub just below, and in between, the toes.

## PROBLEMS WITH DIGESTION AND ELIMINATION

Traveling and business dining are notorious enemies of good digestion and regularity. I find the single most constipating situation in life to be a long flight, where one sits for hours at high altitudes and eats mushy, intestine-blocking food. Fortunately, Aromatherapy helps prevent this problem, even while I'm still in the air. Try these therapeutic self-touches whenever you find yourself in a situation that can cause constipation or indigestion.

### 1. Digestion and Elimination Stimulation

Press the three middle fingers of your right hand into the stomach point, which is located just below the solar plexus, down and over to the right of the liver and gallbladder points. (See Meridian 6 on Diagram 7, page 83, for the exact position.) Then press on both sides of the area between your waist and your thigh to stimulate the colon, using the fingers of both hands. Now press in about four inches below the navel. If any of these points feel sore, go back to the area and press in longer. Wait about an hour after a meal to do these presses.

### 2. Ear Pinches

Diagram 8 on page 88 shows the points to press on the ear for elimination and digestion. Pinch these points on each ear, holding for a count of seven.

### 3. Face Pressures and Pinches

The chin and nose areas relate to the stomach and the colon. (See Diagram 12 on page 152.) Press the cheek on each side of your nose with the first two fingers of each hand. Then gently move the fingers up and down; push the skin, don't slide over it. Repeat ten times. Now pinch the end of your nose. (If you're in a crowded place, you can pretend you are blowing it.) Hold it for six counts, then let go. Repeat three times. Move down to the chin and pinch the middle with the thumb and first finger. Hold for six counts, and repeat three times.

### 4. Arm Pressures

The large intestine meridian runs down the outside of the arm in a direct line from the index finger. (See Diagram 7.) Its most sensitive point is on the forearm, just after the elbow crease. You will find a mound of flesh marking this point, which you should push into with your thumb. Move your thumb around in the point to get a strong reaction. Many people are sore here, which means there is probably blocked-up waste material in the intestine.

The small intestine meridian runs from the little finger up along the inside of the arm. Press small intestine points above the wrist, at the mid-forearm, and at the elbow. All of the intestine presses should be done three times.

### 5. Hand Pinches

The colon and stomach reflex points are located across the middle of the palm. Pinch and press your way across the hand, moving from below the little finger to above the thumb pad, pausing for a count of four each time you pinch. Repeat on both hands three times. (See Diagram 10 on page 95.)

### 6. Foot Points

The key points for the stomach and the colon can be found on the foot chart (Diagram 9 on page 93). To stimulate the small intestine, use your knuckles to rub back and forth on the center of your heels, going in as deeply as possible. To stimulate the colon, start at the "waistline" of each foot (the center arch) and massage in circles back to the heel. Repeat three times. The stomach point is almost halfway down the foot directly below the big toe.

Push into it with your thumb and hold for a count of seven, then release. Repeat three times.

### *TENSION*

Aromatherapy is an excellent remedy for a case of the uptights. The massage zeroes in on ruffled nerve centers and the fragrances uplift the psyche. When everything seems to be going wrong—you've burnt your toast, missed your train, or spent the day arguing with your boss—rub a drop of a calming oil, like lavender, basil, or neroli, into your hands and press the following tension points.

### *1. Solar Plexus Focus*

The main nerves travel through the solar plexus. Focus on calming this area to tranquilize your entire being. Using the left hand (the calming hand, according to polarity theory), make counterclockwise circles over the solar plexus. Even if you are dressed, the motion and warmth of your hand will help to balance your nervous system. (In Chapter 6, on the aroma bath, I describe another way to massage this area, using essential oil—page 130.) After a minute of circling, place your left hand on the center of the solar plexus and cover it with your right hand. Now you are projecting a double energy into the tense area. Close your eyes, think calm thoughts, and hold this position for another minute.

### *2. Back-of-the-Neck and Shoulder Massage*

A common target for tension in the body is the back of the neck and shoulders. Tension makes this area stiff and painful. Dig deeply into the muscles and tendons, following the instructions in Movement 10 under "Wake-Up Massage" (page 89). You will be able to feel the little knots and lactic acid crystals that tension builds, especially when you work at a desk all day. You can give yourself relief even while you are working by massaging your neck and shoulders for three minutes several times a day.

### *FATIGUE*

There are times when all of us succumb to fatigue, and don't have the time for a good night's sleep or a peaceful nap. Aromatherapy can revive you.

Heat some aromatics in your warmer or on a bulb, and rub some into your skin if possible. Stimulating the following energy points will increase your energy.

### 1. Top-of-the-Head Touches

With your fingers and thumbs facing each other, make small firm circles all over the head and on the top of the forehead. Do not slide over the scalp and skin; move it with your fingers. This stimulates the glands and provides a systemic pickup. Repeat three times.

### 2. Solar Plexus Rub

Using the *right* hand (the energizing hand), make counterclockwise circles on the solar plexus. This action will rev up your main nerves, including the vagus nerve that communicates with the brain. Do this for one minute.

### 3. Hand Pressures

Consult the hand chart (Diagram 10 on page 95) and locate the thyroid and adrenal points in the center of your hand. These are two key points that affect your energy. Press these on each hand, holding for a count of seven and releasing. Repeat three times.

### 4. Foot Work

The feet are vital sources of energy, and can be good friends or thieving enemies. Pressures from bad shoes can give you a headache and tire you quickly. By massaging the feet with caring hands you can revive every nerve center in the body. Be sure that your shoes fit and give your feet ample support. Press and work your feet often, especially if you've spent long hours on them. Consult the foot chart (Diagram 9 on page 93) for important positions and let your fingers do the walking. When you are tired, focus on the thyroid and adrenal points, which are located on the metatarsal pad; pressing them will send energizing messages all the way to the top of your head. Remember that all important body functions—blood, lymph, and nerve endings—travel up from the feet and back down again.

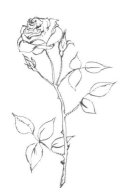

*V*

# *THE LOVING TOUCH*

Most of us believe that the most profound knowledge of another person comes to us through the intensity of sex. Although sex does give us rapid access to another person's body and mind, there is more to be learned by touch than sex alone can teach us. Sex is one of the most intimate acts two people can share, but it can also be one of the most private. During the high-voltage lovemaking experience, you are swept full force into the tumult of your own physical sensations, which makes it difficult for you to concentrate on your partner's body and feelings. For better or worse, it is possible to make love without ever fully comprehending what passion *feels* like to your partner, and it is only the most sensitive and accomplished lovers who can tune into and tap their mate's deepest sensual responses—a sad truth, which often makes sex more pleasurable for one partner than the other.

Aromatherapy can give you a new and better understanding of your lover's body. As you massage the partner who has surrendered himself or herself to your touch, you will strike up a dramatic new acquaintance with the body beneath your hands. Many aspects of this familiar physical landscape will surprise you when you explore it objectively with your fingers. You will note, perhaps for the first time, the parts and pieces of the joints, and the many knobs and niches of the spine. You will feel the texture of your partner's skin, and discover which areas of his bodily terrain are especially strong, ticklish, or sensitive. If your partner is a woman, you will relish the softness of her abdominal curves, and the bounciness and resilience of her buttocks; if he is a man, you will admire the sweep and curve of his muscles.

Through the polarity principles, so essential to Aromatherapy massage, you will learn much about the way your partner's energy complements yours. Once you have defined your lover's body with your hands, you will have more feeling for it. As you and your partner exchange scentual touch, you will help each other to feel more comfortable with your naked selves, and reduce some of the shyness and lack of confidence all of us have about our bodies. Scentual touch also provides a transition between everyday routine and the intense, emotional sexual climate.

Scentual massage results in increased sensuous awareness, and inspires deeper and franker communication in all areas of love. When you translate the lessons of scentual touch into sensual passion, your capacity for sexual pleasure will greatly expand.

## SCENTUAL ATTRACTION

The essential oils emphasize and enhance the attraction that our natural odors inspire in one another. All living species—animals, insects, and plants—exude scented secretions that attract and repel. These odoriferous chemical compounds, called *pheromones*, act as warning signals, territory markers, or mating calls. The queen bee, for example, uses her pheromone to keep the other ladies of the hive from becoming sexually mature and competing for the throne. The boar can freeze his sow in the mating position by giving her a whiff of his sexual perfume. Scientists are just beginning to understand the way human pheromones affect relationships between people. A study conducted by the University of Birmingham in England revealed that men exposed to androstenol, a steroid in underarm perspiration, found photographs of normally dressed women far more attractive than did a control group, which did not sniff the pheromone. Research at the University of Chicago showed that women who lived together in dormitories eventually had closely timed menstrual cycles, due to their mutual response to the odor of glandular secretions. Subtle but potent odors also encourage or discourage us to relate to one another. The pheromones of potential mates are registered through a *vomeronasal organ* in the roof of the nasal cavity, and romance either is born or dies. Most of us, however, remain unaware of how our sense of smell influences our passions. We may be attracted or put off by the way others smell, yet be completely unconscious that they have any smell at all. We may attribute our unmistakable feelings of allure to our lover's soft skin, curly hair, or perfect shape, when, in fact, it is his unique sexual fragrance that beckons.

Perfumers of the world—from ancient alchemists to modern scent makers—have exploited the ability of fragrance to inspire romance. Cleopatra, one of history's most desirable women, well understood the power of perfume. She floated down the Nile into Anthony's arms wreathed in fragrance; not only was her body rubbed with irresistible essential oils, but the very sails of her ship were soaked in them. As Cleopatra and her perfumer knew,

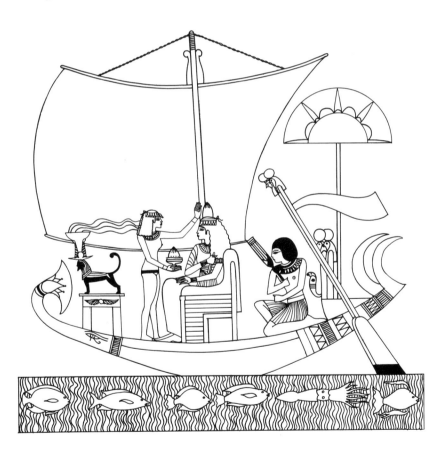

natural scents are the most erotic. Essential oils are nothing more or less than concentrated plant pheromones—sweet scents that attract pollinators— and they seem to draw humans to one another as they draw the bee and hummingbird to the fragrant blossom. All woods, roots, and flowers produce eros-stimulating essences; some, like patchouli, ylang-ylang, and jasmine, are renowned for their erotic lure. Unfortunately, those of us who want nature's pheromones on our own vanity tables today must go to some effort to obtain and mix the pure, unadulterated essential oils. Most modern perfumes, with their large percentages of synthetic fragrances, are not nearly as devastating as the old-fashioned scents of the thirties and forties, like Shalimar, that transported the admirers of Gloria Swanson and Greta Garbo to Shangri-la.

## LOVE IN THE AIR

With the intriguing powers of scent in mind, create a fragrant atmosphere to begin your scentual massage. For a calming, uplifting, and romantic aura, heat a quality essential oil in the room where you plan to reexplore your partner's body. Ylang-ylang, jasmine and patchouli, oil of sandalwood, rose, cinnamon, and cedarwood are all eros-inspiring. A drop of naturally volatile essence on a warm lightbulb, or in a specially designed heater, will soon fill the room with sensual fragrance. Be sure not to heat the oil at too high a temperature, because overheated oils quickly evaporate. Coordinate your room fragrance with your massage oil to double the essence impact. Be sure to use more of the essence in the room than in the massage oil (see Appendix I) to prevent your scent message from being diluted when the oils are exposed to the air.

## SENSUAL TOUCHES

Even the basic massage (outlined in Chapter III) can be erotically arousing when performed by lovers in the nude in intimately lit and scentual surroundings. But for even greater sensuality, you will want to use the special strokes and polarity presses that concentrate on parts of the body that are sexually responsive.

Most of us think the genitals and nipples are the only libidinous parts of the body, but actually the ears, hands, feet, solar plexus, and neck are all erogenous zones. These areas contain nerve endings or are meridian centers, and they strongly affect hormone- and energy-producing glands. Since stimulating hormones and body energy create sexual response and drive, caressing and stroking these sex-sensitive areas will not only make your partner swoon with momentary pleasure, but will initiate long-lasting passion. You will use a variety of strokes on the erotic areas, from firm and deep to light and feathery.

### 1. Ear Touch

Taking one ear at a time, gently pinch all around it with your forefinger and thumb, working from the outside in. Then take your forefinger and *very* lightly trace around the entire ear area, from the outside to the center. Now do both ears at the same time, using the right and left fingers. End with your fingers in both ears, and hold them there for a few seconds, vibrating them slightly. Consult the ear chart on page 88 to make sure that you are touching the adrenal gland, sexual organ, and sense points at the lower inside of the ear and on the lobe during the pinching process.

### 2. Hand Touch

Grasp one of your partner's hands in both of yours and stroke it, pulling from the top of the hand out to the end of the fingertips. Then, holding the hand in one of yours, massage each finger with the thumb and first three fingers of your other hand. Work from the base of the finger to the tip, and then give the finger a firm pull. The tip of the thumb contains the brain/pituitary meridian and an extra pinch here wakes up your partner's energy. Finally, very lightly stroke the inside of the palm with your fingers and repeat the process on your partner's other hand. Refer to the hand chart on page 95 and zero in on the adrenal point at mid-hand and the sexual organ point on the wrist, just below the thumb side of the hand.

### 3. Toe Touch

The bottoms of the feet and toes are wildly sensitive, an advantage and disadvantage during scentual touch. If you bear down on blocked meridian points too hard, your partner will experience more pain than pleasure. On the other hand, if you stroke too lightly you can tickle your partner off the table. Take your touch cue from your partner's reaction. Your partner should lie face up or sit in a chair with feet propped up. Start by standing at the end of the massage table or kneeling at the end of the body (if on the floor), or sit at the propped-up feet (if your partner is sitting). With both hands run your thumbs up the feet as you do in the basic massage (Movement 40, Illustration III–27). Then, taking one foot at a time, work on each toe, massaging each one with kneading and stroking motions, and finishing with an emphatic pull. The big toe contains important gland points, so be sure to give it your concentration. Then, referring to the foot chart on page 93, press the adrenal and sexual organ points and hold for a count of seven. Finish by stroking each foot in both hands five times, and holding the flat of your hands on both feet for twenty counts. Since your partner is lying face up or is seated, you will be putting your right hand on his left foot, and your left hand on his right foot, transmitting an energizing polarity charge.

### 4. Neck Touch

Orientals have always regarded a woman's neck as an erogenous zone. In old Chinese and Japanese paintings a woman's body is concealed by a gorgeous kimono, but the provocative curve of her neck is sensuously bare. I believe we should pay more attention to our necks, from an aesthetic, sensual, and therapeutic point of view. Main arteries, nerves, and lymph all course through the neck. As you will discover, it is also unusually sensitive to touch. With your partner lying face up, use the basic massage techniques that affect the neck. (See Chapter III, Movements 16, 35, and 36.) For a provocative addition, stroke upward from the top of the shoulders to the base of the skull with a feather-light touch, starting from the inside and working out to the ears. Repeat this move at least five times. Then, placing the first and second fingers of both hands at the base of the skull (the occipital bone), make little feathery circles, working from the center of the head to the ears and back. Do this five times, or until your partner begs you to stop because it feels so good.

### 5. Solar Plexus Touch

The word *solar* means "sun" (and its warming energy) and *plexus* means "a grouping." The solar plexus, situated between the breastbone and the navel, is a vital energy center and extraordinarily sensitive. The vagus nerve, a cranial nerve that affects many organs, runs from the base of the brain through the solar plexus and ends in the abdominal cavity. Because the solar plexus is a center of feeling, it is too sensitive to be deeply pressed during massage. For this reason, polarity is a wonderfully effective technique for this area. The stimulating force of your positive right hand can energize your partner when you lay it flat, with the fingers pointed toward the head, on the solar plexus, for a count of twenty. Hold your partner's right arm with your left hand while you do this. If your partner needs calming, lay your left hand on the solar plexus and hold his left arm with your right hand. To balance the entire system, slip the right hand under your partner's back, directly under the solar plexus, and hold the left hand on the solar plexus as described above. With this move you are creating a connecting current and stimulating the solar plexus between your hands. The trick is to hold each of these positions until your partner begins to feel a vital life force coursing through his body.

### POLARITY PRESSES

During the highly charged lovemaking process, you are most apt to feel the electrical currents that flow through your body, and how they can be transmitted—and received—by another human being. This mysterious but very real charge is a form of electromagnetic energy, which has been known by various names for thousands of years. Hippocrates called it "Vis Medicatrix Naturae" (Nature's life force); Indian yogis call it "prana"; and the Chinese term it "chi." Recently modern scientists have found that there is an electromagnetic field in each of our cells that ceases to function only when we do. A special photographic process developed at Duke University proved that the electrical charges people produce register as a halo outside of the body. It is this charge, too, that shows up on a lie detector test, and can give us small shocks in the winter.

Therapeutic polarity touches make use of this vital life current and can put you and your partner in touch with each other's electrical charges. Because the following electromagnetic presses enable you to stimulate each other's vital life forces, they are an excellent prelude to making love. At first you may feel as if nothing is happening. Don't be discouraged; remember, it takes time and practice before you get the hang of the moves. Eventually you will experience the unique sensation of activated energy. The more calm and collected you and your partner are, the better polarity will work.

### DOUBLE PRESSES

Here are several polarity presses that you and your partner can do to each other at the same time.

### 1. Sandwich Press

This body-on-body seductive press is deceptively simple, but very effective. The lightest partner should lie on top of the heaviest, stretching out full length and matching limb to limb. Both your heads are turned to the side. (See Illustration V–1.) Both partners must totally let go of tension and restraint; the person on the bottom should sink into the floor, and the person

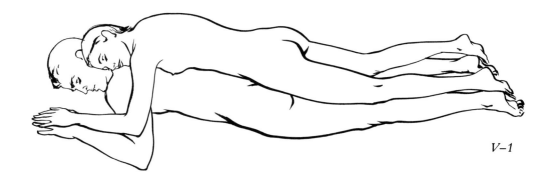

V–1

on top should try to meld into him. This weird and wonderful position supplies electrical grounding for the bottom partner, and the partner on top is buoyed up, as though he's lying on a living mattress. The press is seductive, but also therapeutic, stimulating the spinal nerves of the bottom partner with the solar plexus nerve center of the partner on top, and vice versa.

### 2. Back-to-Back Press

Sit back to back on the floor with your partner. (See Illustration V–2.) Press as deeply as you can into one another; feel your spines communicating, exchanging warmth and vital energy. This press stimulates the spinal nerves that communicate with the brain and organs. Hold for a count of ten, lean forward for a moment, then return and hold for another ten counts.

### 3. Neck-to-Neck Press

Sit back to back with your buttocks pushed forward enough so that each partner can put his head on the other's shoulder. (See Illustration V–3.) Hold for a count of ten, then reverse positions and hold for ten again. (See Illustration V–4.) This affectionate pose creates a quiet but meaningful unity, and helps relieve neck and shoulder tension.

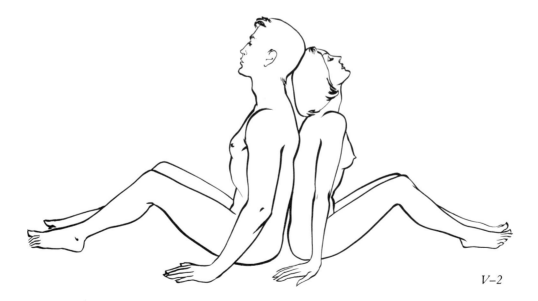

*V–2*

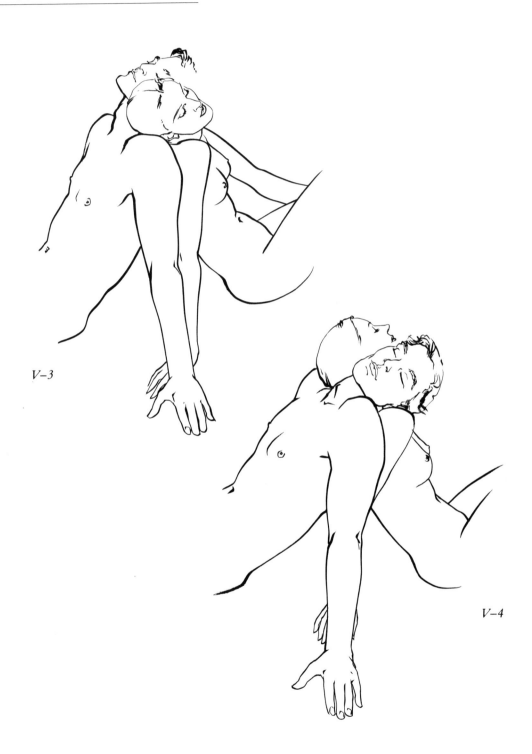

V–3

V–4

*EXCHANGE PRESSES*

Do the following series of presses to your partner, then change positions and have your partner do them to you. Remember that the basic polarity principles are similar to the rules of electricity: two negatives repel, and two positives attract. In polarity, the left side of the body is negative and the right is positive. The flat left hand is calming, and the flat right hand is stimulating. The fingers stir up energy. Before beginning, boost your conductability by rubbing your hands briskly together. This will send you well-charged into the massage. Think of using yourself as a conduit for your partner's energy, instead of putting your own energy into your partner.

### 1. Soothing Shoulder Press

Your partner should lie face up on the floor, while you kneel next to your partner's shoulders. Press down firmly on both shoulders with your hands. (See Illustration V–5.) Hold for a count of ten. This reduces tension in the neck and shoulder area.

### 2. Collarbone Press

With your partner lying face up, press with your fingers on the collarbone (or clavicle). (See Illustration V–6.) This is a lymph point and pressing it helps drain the body of libido-inhibiting toxins. Hold for a count of ten.

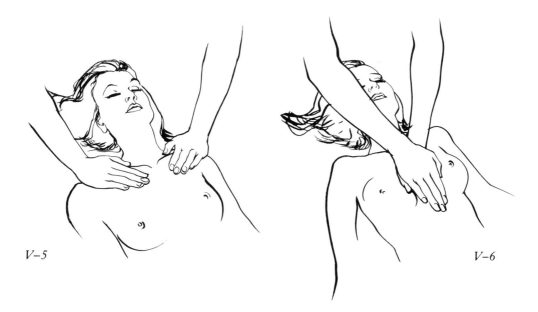

V–5                                                                V–6

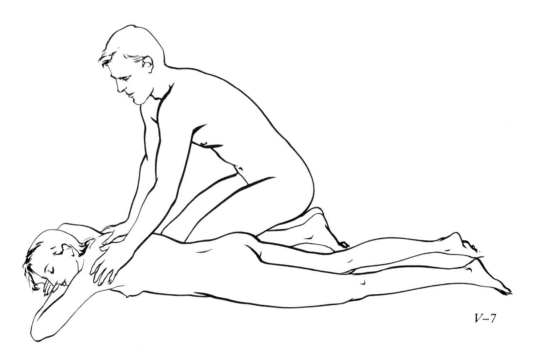

V–7

### 3. Stimulating Shoulder Blade Press

Have your partner turn over and lie face down; then press with your fingers just at the base of the shoulder blades. (See Illustration V–7.) This helps relieve upper back tension and stimulates the heart-lung meridians. Hold for ten counts.

### 4. Happy Hand Press

To establish a warm feeling of contact between you and your partner, kneel above your partner and reach down to the hands, which are lying palms up at your partner's side. (See Illustration V–8.) Fit your hand into your part-ner's hand and press, holding for ten counts. This is a general stimulant for all the mid-body organs and adrenal glands.

### 5. Straddle Press

Straddle your partner and press on the lower half of the buttocks with both hands. Hold the pressure for ten counts. (See Illustration V–9.) Important

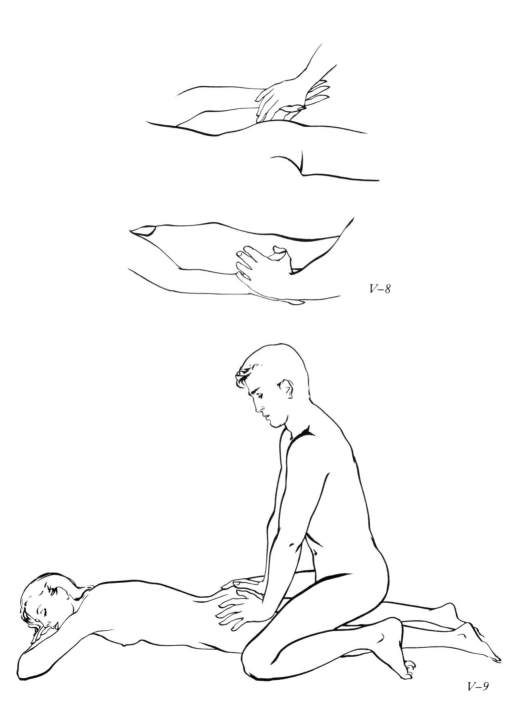

V-8

V-9

nerves cross over this area, which relate to the woman's uterus and the man's groin. While you are still straddling the body, move down and press the thighs and ankles for ten counts to stimulate the bladder meridian.

### 6. Foot-to-Foot Press

Your partner should lie face down and you should stand with your back to your partner. With your heels "walk" on the front part of the bottom of your partner's feet, alternating your weight from foot to foot. (You can balance your weight by holding on to something.) Gently move into a position where your arches meet. (See Illustration V–10.) Hold only as long as it is comfortable for the pressed partner, then change positions, and let your partner walk on your feet. This move, stimulating to important glands and organs (see foot chart on page 93), should be approached with sensitivity and care.

### 7. Top-of-the-Shoulder Press

Sit your partner in a straight chair, with feet on the floor and arms at the sides. Standing behind, lean over and press your forearms down on the top of the shoulders. Put as much pressure as you can into the press without

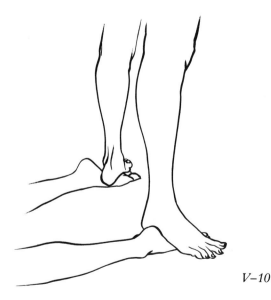

V–10

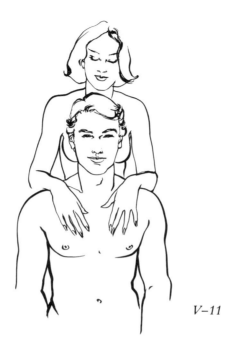

*V–11*

hurting your partner. (See Illustration V–11.) This relieves tension buildup in the neck and shoulders.

### 8. Mystical Brain Balancing

This move will help your partner "get his head together" for love, and focused on you after a tough day. It uses the natural energy in the head and hands to synchronize brain currents. Put your right hand behind his head at the base of the skull, and the left hand over the forehead. (See Illustration V–12.) Hold for a count of twenty, encouraging your partner to let go of inhibiting tensions, eyes closed, torso relaxed, letting the body's natural electricity get to work. Try to relax yourself, too.

### 9. Energizing Back Body Sweep

Your partner should sit on a stool, back straight and arms at the sides. Stand behind the stool and starting at the top of the shoulders, sweep the hands down to the opposite buttock, crossing mid-back. Hold your hands about

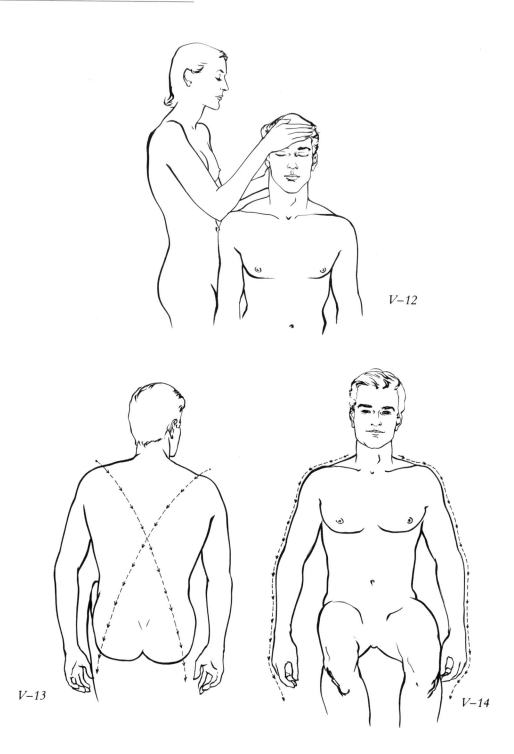

V–12

V–13

V–14

one inch out from the body, and sweep in one motion, quickly with assurance. Repeat three times. (See Illustration V–13.) As with all of the polarity techniques in this book, although this move does not touch your partner, your body's own electromagnetic energy will affect your partner's. This movement will energize and revitalize.

### 10. Calming Front Body Sweep

Stand in front of your partner, who is seated as before. Lean over and sweep your hands from the base of the neck, across the shoulders and down over the hands. (See Illustration V–14.) Again, hold your hands one inch away from the body and do not actually touch your partner. This is a calming, balancing move, which should be done more slowly than the back sweep. Repeat three times.

### 11. Balancing Full Body Sweep

As you have seen by the previous two moves, a polarity body sweep can either calm or energize, depending on the direction and speed you use. If your partner is tense and nervous you will want to sweep the energy slowly from the head to the feet. To recharge a fatigued partner, sweep slowly from the feet to the head. (See Illustration V–15.) Your partner should be lying face up and your hands should just skim the body. Do these sweeps three times, always in the same direction.

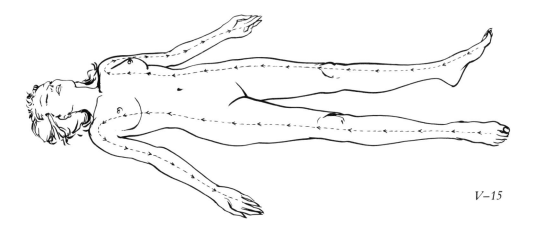

*V–15*

## ___HELLO-GOODBYE MASSAGE_____

You do not always have to set aside a special time and place for scentual touch; massage can also become an integral part of the everyday routine you share with your mate. A touching goodbye at the door should help you both face the stress and energy-taxing tasks that await you; an affectionate, therapeutic hello at the end of the day can be more relaxing and reviving than a drink and cigarette.

Try to incorporate the following stimulating touches into your life.

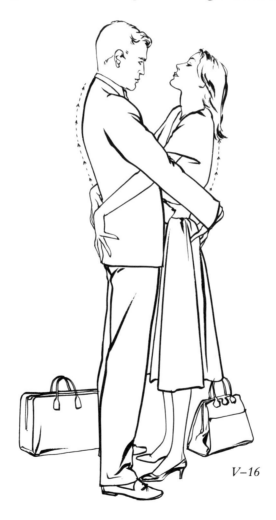

V–16

### 1. Vertical Massage

Standing toe to toe you should both place the fingers of both of your hands on either side of the base of each other's spines. (This is the sacral area.) (See Illustration V–16.) Press deeply on either side of the spine and run your fingers all the way up to the base of one another's skulls. Return your hands to starting position and repeat six times. This simple massage activates the nervous system—necessary before or after a tiring day.

### 2. Cheek-to-Cheek Massage

Embrace warmly and stand cheek to cheek. This massage move may look like the fox trot, but it stimulates the stomach, bowels, digestion, lungs, sinuses, eyes, and nose. Circle your cheek around your partner's cheek five times on each side. (See Illustration V–17.)

### 3. Eskimo Kiss Massage

While you are still embracing, take the opportunity to rub noses with your partner. The nose is a stomach-digestion meridian, and is lined with the same erectile tissue found in sexual organs, which makes it extremely sensitive. (During sex, the nostrils may expand, causing the tissue to swell. If this happens too often the nasal lining can become blocked; doctors call this condition "honeymoon nose.") It may be better to say hello instead of good-bye with a nose rub, as this massage move could make you late for work.

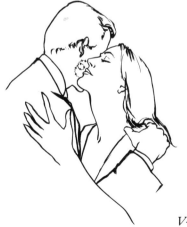

*V–17*

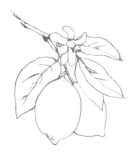

*VI*

# THE AROMA BATH

The aroma bath is an important part of your Aromatherapy program for health and beauty. This unique bathing system includes morning and night routines—a combination of massage, water, and essential oils—as well as special baths for fun and therapy.

## THE HISTORY OF BATHS

Before you turn your bathroom into a restorative spa, consider your physiological relationship to water. Scientists believe that the first living creatures crawled up out of primordial seas; our present-day bodies, composed mainly of water, mirror the chemical structure of seawater in their life-maintaining fluids. Because the fetus is gestated in a salty, mineralized "bath" that cushions the fetus in the womb, we still "crawl" from a protective and soothing watery environment to a drier—and harsher—reality.

For these reasons, perhaps, bathing is one of our most natural impulses. Man has always worshipped water as the very source of life and made baths a religious and personal ritual. Mythology is filled with gods, nymphs, and water sprites who reside in oceans, rivers, lakes, and streams. Since ancient times, religious ceremonies of purification and rebirth have included bathing.

Bathing has also always been a pleasurable activity. Sumptuous bathrooms with primitive drainage systems have been found in Egyptian and Indian excavations, dating back to 4,000 B.C. No ancient culture, however, rivaled the Romans for balneal enthusiasm.

These pleasure-loving conquerors bathed their way across the world, from

Britain to Africa. Bathing for the Romans was a way to socialize and entertain themselves, as well as to get scrupulously clean. Some of the public baths, like those at Caracella, built in A.D. 217, could wash two thousand bodies at a time. As the hedonistic Romans became ever more decadent, public bathing began to include a bit of wet and slippery sex.

The Roman bathing ritual was the first to incorporate elements of the Aromatherapy bath. After entering the "thermae," or bathing room, the bather was undressed and rubbed with fragrant essential oils. He exercised to work up a sweat, then, in a steam room, had his skin scraped down to smoothness with a metal instrument, which cleansed his pores. After that he was massaged, rinsed off, soaked in warm water, and refreshed by an icy plunge. The final stop in this five-hour moisture marathon was the Unctuarium, where rare and costly perfumes were applied in a fragrant rubdown.

Though even the most beauty-conscious moderns haven't the time to indulge in five-hour baths today, the Romans had the right idea. Baths are the first step to skin beauty, because water softens the skin more than any other element. You can prove this to yourself by soaking your hand in plain vegetable oil; the skin will look more or less the same after this process as it did before. Soak your hand in plain water, however, and you will see the skin turn white and wrinkle, as the water softens it and changes its structure. The softening effect of the water enables smoothing oils to penetrate the skin more easily, and seal in the revitalizing moisture the water has supplied. Since different essential oils have different effects on both the skin and the nerves, the Aromatherapy combination of water, massage, and essential oils can detoxify, deodorize, and soften the skin, correct skin imbalances, promote new cell growth, and revitalize and calm the nervous system. The essential oils that you will use to scent the air, water, and yourself will provide you with a wide variety of bathing experiences—from seriously therapeutic to playfully sexy.

## THE DRY BRUSH MASSAGE

Dry brushing is a form of self-massage that is widely practiced in bath-oriented countries, like Norway and Sweden. Because dry brushing is a stimulating process that helps rid your skin of the dead cells it sheds during the night, and improves blood and lymph circulation, you will probably want to do it before your morning bath or shower. Dry brushing can be done, however, before the evening bath you take to prepare yourself for a special occasion, when you want to glow with increased vitality.

### The Equipment

You will need a natural-bristle body brush, preferably one with a detachable long handle that can be used when brushing your back. These are available at bath supply stores and health food stores. If your brush hasn't got a handle, a flat loofah with a loop at each end will also bring your back into reachable range. Soft natural bristles and a flat loofah are better for your skin than a brush with nylon bristles, which have a tendency to scratch. However, if your skin is sensitive and dry, take it easy with even a soft, natural-bristle brush, especially in winter. Gauge the force of your brushing by the way it feels: you should be glowing, not bleeding.

It is important to keep your brush or loofah clean, since it is lifting off dead skin and impurities. Wash it in mild soap or detergent, rinse well, and towel dry. It will need a full day to dry thoroughly before the next bath. Don't wash natural bristles in water that's too hot, or the bristles will weaken.

### The Brushing Technique

Rub exactly *one drop* of your favorite essential oil into your brush to add a delightful scent to the brushing process. Start by brushing your feet: hold on to the wall or a piece of furniture with one hand, and brush with the other. Brush your soles, toes, tops of feet, and ankles. Do one foot at a time, then work your way up your legs, brushing from ankle to thigh. Concentrate on the pad at the outer top of your thigh (see Illustration VI–1), where cellulite gathers, especially in women. Cellulite is toxic tissue that collects water and fat in little clumps, making the skin look like the peel of an orange. It is unhealthy and unsightly, and can be improved by rigorous dry brushing, and bathing and massaging with essential oils. (See the recipe for treating cellulite in Appendix I.)

Now move to your hands and brush the tops, fingers, and palms. Brush on up the arm, moving all around and paying special attention to your

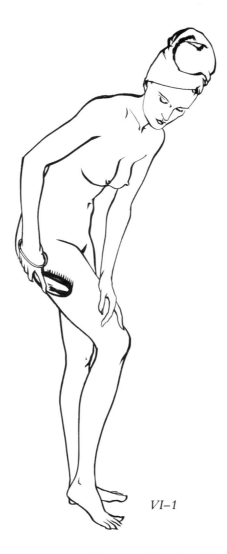

VI–1

elbows, which have a tendency to become discolored, rough, and scaly. After finishing your arms, brush across the tops of your shoulders and the back of the neck. For those who are developing a fat pad, or "hump," on the back of the neck, brushing in small circles all over and around the area helps to reduce congestion and tension.

Now you are ready to begin dry brushing the torso. Brush lightly across the chest, a sensitive area. Do not brush the breasts or nipples, as they are too sensitive for this process. Move down to the solar plexus and brush it in small circles, moving from the right to the left side. If you have large breasts that interfere with the brushing, hold them up with one hand. Continue on around the abdomen, still brushing in circles. Move the brush in a clockwise pattern to stimulate colon activity as well as to reduce any fat you may be harboring between your waist and pelvis.

Starting at the right side of your waist, brush in small circles around the top of your hip and over the right buttock. You can really have a good go at this area, since it's mostly fat and not very sensitive. Repeat on the other side. To brush your back put the handle in your brush, or use the flat loofah. Beginning at the top of your shoulders, work back and forth over your entire back down to the top of your legs. Be careful to avoid any moles you might have on your back—or anywhere else, for that matter—don't brush directly on them, since you might tear them, and moles are temperamental and not to be tampered with. You should be glowing all over by now, and ready for your Aromatherapy bath or shower.

## THE BATHS

The following baths incorporate methods used by the Japanese and Scandinavians as well as by European Aromatherapists. All of these bathing techniques should give you pleasure while they improve your health and the quality of your skin. In all of the following baths, the basic idea is to clean first, then stimulate and restore.

Take a hint from the Japanese, who clean themselves *before* they get into a tub of water. If you wash before you bathe you will not be "stewing in your own juice," and the goodness of the oils and herbs you put into the water can work unimpeded by body impurities and soap. Take a shower, or, if you haven't got one, do a quick body wash with a washcloth while standing in your tub. Soap your genitals, and rinse thoroughly. Then begin to fill the tub based on the instructions given for one of the baths that follow.

*THE RELAXING BATH*

A relaxing bath is a body and soul refresher, best taken at the end of a hectic day, when you want to go forth into the evening refreshed, collected, and delightfully fragrant. If you are preparing for bed, this soothing bath will help you sleep like a baby.

1. After cleaning yourself, begin to fill the tub with water that feels warmer than your hand, but not very hot. The temperature should be about 98 degrees Fahrenheit. As the tub fills, add either 10 drops of essential oil, a capful of an aromatic bath oil you have bought or prepared, or herbs wrapped and tied in a little cloth bag or in a metal tea cage.

    If you are using essential oils, lavender is a super bath-relaxer and can be used alone. Or you can try one of the following oil recipes, which are also calming; they are to be used neat with no carrier oil.

    i. 6 drops of lavender and 4 drops of geranium
    ii. 7 drops of chamomile and 3 drops of basil
    iii. 7 drops of sandalwood and 3 drops of marjoram

    If you are using herbs, the dried herbs can be added in the cloth or tea cage, or in the form of a strong tea (half a cup of herbs to 2 cups of boiling water). Try mixing linden with sage or chamomile with rose. A strong solution of chamomile tea alone is also calming to the skin and nervous system.

    Herbs can be added as you begin to fill the tub, but essential oils should be put in when it is almost full, since they evaporate faster.

2. With your head wrapped in a towel, pinned up, or in a shower cap, stretch out as far as you can so that the water covers as much of your body as possible. Close your eyes and breathe in the relaxing fragrance of the herbs or oils. Feel them seeping into your psyche and into your system. Imagine yourself floating in a calm, peaceful sea as you soak for ten minutes. (If your body seems tense or tight, you may want to do the massage movements described below.)

3. Rise up slowly out of the water, maintaining your sense of calm and feeling of being centered. Hug yourself in a big, soft, luxurious towel.

Following my instructions for applying massage oils after the bath (which appear at the end of this chapter on page 139), stroke on a prepared massage oil, or a calming combination of essential oils you have made yourself. For relaxation and calm, try one of the following recipes, which should be mixed in 4 ounces of carrier oil.

    i. 5 drops of lavender and 3 drops of vetiver
    ii. 6 drops of chamomile and 2 drops of rose
    iii. 5 drops of marjoram and 3 drops of neroli

4. Put on a natural-fiber robe; I like cotton terry, because it absorbs any leftover dampness. If you are bathing in preparation to go out, try to allow yourself fifteen minutes to lie completely flat with no pillow before getting dressed. This post-bath relaxation will give your system time to register the restorative effects of your bath, and to readjust to ordinary room temperature.

## BATH MASSAGE

While you are soaking in your relaxing bath or after you have emerged, you can further unwind with an easy series of therapeutic massage movements.

### 1. Collarbone Sweep

Place the index and third fingers of both hands under the two collarbones below the center of your neck. Slide the fingers all the way to the tips of your shoulders. Repeat six times. (See Illustration VI–2.) This stimulates lymph flow.

### 2. Breast Circle

With your hands placed at the outside of each breast, run the heel of the hand down to the waist. Then come in under the breast with your fingers, and run them up the middle of your chest to your collarbone. Make this continuing circle around each breast six times. (See Illustration VI–3.) This stimulates the lymph and lungs and is good for chest and breast congestion.

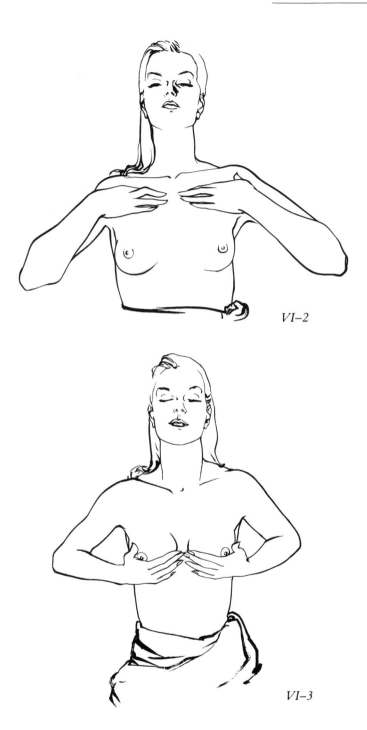

VI–2

VI–3

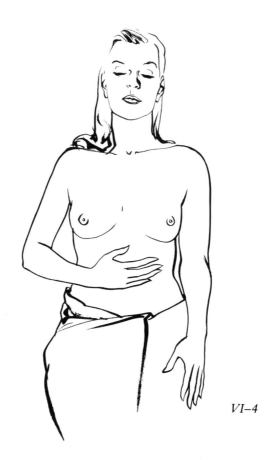

VI–4

### 3. Solar Plexus Talk

When you lie in a tub of warm water, your solar plexus relaxes automatically. This is a great time to really "talk" to it with your hands. Place one hand under your breast, and with the other stroke your solar plexus in a counterclockwise circle. If you need calming use your left hand; if you want a pickup, use the right hand. (See Illustration VI–4.)

### 4. Hand-Arm Squeeze and Slide

Squeeze your hands together in a prayer position. (See Illustration VI–5.) Then, maintaining your squeezing grip, slide your right hand up the left arm all the way to the shoulder. Work with squeezing strokes all the way around the arm. Repeat, using the left hand on the right arm. (See Illustration VI–6.) This stimulates digestive and intestinal points, and relieves stiffness or tension in the arms and hands.

### 5. Leg Slide Strokes

Lean back and balance your body on your forearms. Bring up one knee, leaving your foot flat on the bottom of the tub. Place the other leg over the drawn-up knee, resting it at the ankle. Then press the top leg down as hard

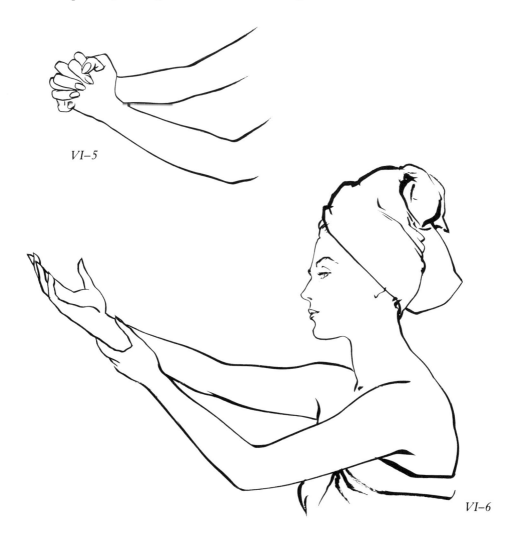

VI–5

VI–6

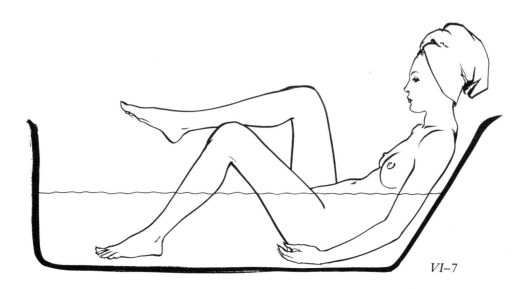

VI–7

as you can on your supporting knee, and slide it from the ankle up along the calf to the back of the top knee. (See Illustration VI–7.) Repeat six times for each leg, going back to the ankle and up to the knee, massaging the back of the top leg as deeply as possible. This stimulates sexual organs and the bladder meridian, and refreshes tired legs.

### 6. Limbic-stimulating Lumbar Stretch

Warm water loosens up tight muscles, including those in the lower back, where many of us feel painful tension. Stretching the lower back (the lumbar area) works well in a relaxing bath. Be sure you move slowly, feeling your way to a comfortable stretch, which you should hold for a count of five at first, and then, as time goes on, for a count of ten. Bring your knees up, feet flat on the bottom of the tub, about a foot apart. Lean forward from the *hip*, rounding the back slightly, with your arms stretched toward the toes. (See Illustration VI–8.) Breathe deeply, inhaling the aromatics you have added to the tub. You are not only stretching your back, you are also turning on your limbic system via your sense of smell, and giving yourself a physiological and psychological lift.

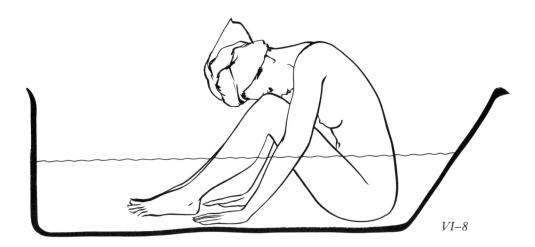

*VI–8*

## THE STIMULATING BATH

A stimulating bath is the perfect activity for days and evenings when you need a pickup that is neither addicting nor fattening. This bath increases circulation, revs up the adrenal glands, and as a result helps reduce weight and cellulite.

1. First, dry brush your body according to the instructions at the beginning of this chapter.
2. Wash yourself, then half fill the tub with water that feels only tepid to the touch. The hotter the water, the more relaxing; the cooler, the more stimulating. Add one of the following recipes of stimulating oils:

     I. 7 drops of juniper and 3 drops of basil
     II. 5 drops of rosemary and 5 drops of geranium
     III. 4 drops of rosemary, 4 drops of juniper, and 2 drops of peppermint

The following herbs, alone or in the suggested combinations, also make effective bathing stimulants.

     I. Rosemary, peppermint, and comfrey root
     II. Lemongrass, savory, and basil

Swish whatever aromatics you choose around in the water, then get in the tub. Using a large washcloth, briskly rub the water all over your body.

3. Take the plug out of the tub and start running in cold water. Mix the cold and warm water with your hands until you are sitting in water as cold as you can stand it. Put the plug back in and swish the cold water all over yourself, dunking your body down into it several times. Then step out of the tub.

4. The most stimulating way to dry yourself is to slap yourself dry with your hands. This is a version of a Scandinavian custom, in which the wet body is slapped dry with twigs. Begin slapping your arms and legs, then move over to the back of the neck, then on to the chest. With both hands beat on your solar plexus, telling it to wake up. Slap over your stomach, hips, and buttocks until they are pink, then continue slapping your thighs, lower legs, and feet. (See Illustration VI–9.) Keep your hands loose and relaxed as you slap; the slaps should provide a reawakening tingle, but should not be painful.

5. Rub yourself hard all over with a textured terry towel. A special friction-ribbed towel will prove the most stimulating. True bathing enthusiasts open the window, even in winter, and run in place for one minute, breathing deeply as the invigorating air circulates around their nude bodies. Try it for an extra glow, but be careful not to let the North winds chill you.

6. Finish your bath by massaging your body with one of the following essential-oil stimulating recipes mixed in 4 ounces of carrier oil.

   i. 3 drops of rosemary, 3 drops of lavender, and 2 drops of geranium
   ii. 3 drops of juniper, 3 drops of lavender, and 2 drops of eucalyptus

## THE VIRTUES OF THE COLD RINSE

Members of the nation's Polar Bear clubs have a beauty secret. A cold rinse, after any bath, is a skin beautifier. When you douse the skin in cold water the hair follicles contract. The important nerves surrounding these pores are stimulated during the contraction process. Since these nerves are partly responsible for cell production, stimulating them helps produce new cells,

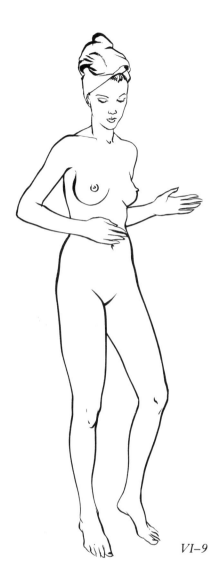

VI–9

which, of course, give your skin a more youthful and vital look. In my
opinion, too many people damage their skin by using very hot water in
their baths and showers, which dries the outer layer and breaks little red
capillaries just beneath the surface. Cold water is also a good diet aid, since
it speeds up the metabolism.

*THE SCENTUAL BATH*

A soothing, warm, aromatic bath with romantic essences and herbs relaxes your mind and body, and puts all your senses on alert, preparing them for the erotic experience. The voluptuous fragrances travel up through your olfactory system, into the seat of emotions, exciting memories of past love and providing a sensuous atmosphere for the present. You can reinforce the scentual effect by burning the same oils in the bedroom that you use in your bath and on your body. You may want to try the following bath alone, or with a lover.

1. Run warm water halfway into the tub, and add the essential oils, the herbs, or a good-quality prepared bath oil. Then finish filling the tub. If you are using essential oil, try one of these combinations:

    i. 4 drops of patchouli, 3 drops of lavender, and 2 drops of rose
    ii. 4 drops of ylang-ylang, 2 drops of vetiver, and 3 drops of geranium

    The leaves and petals of flowers make marvelous scentual bath aromatics. If you have a garden, you may want to dry the petals for a yearlong potpourri. Rose, honeysuckle, lily, and carnation petals can be used fresh, and geranium leaves, lavender, and clover are lovely when dried.

2. Soak for five minutes and then massage your arms and legs with upward strokes. Circle your solar plexus in a clockwise direction, talking to it, and telling it this is going to be a romantic evening. If your lover has joined you in the bath, you may want to practice some of your massage moves on his feet, neck, and shoulders.

3. Step out of the tub and gently pat yourself (or your partner) dry. Stroke on a scentual oil, reveling in its nourishing fragrance. In 4 ounces of carrier oil, try:

    i. 3 drops of patchouli, 2 drops of lavender, and 2 drops of sandalwood
    ii. 3 drops of ylang-ylang, 2 drops of basil, and 2 drops of sandalwood

*THERAPEUTIC BATHS*

If you are really ill, running a fever, or nauseated, it is best not to take a full bath; simply sponge off underarms and genitals. However, a therapeutic bath can do much to speed your recovery if you are suffering from a stuffy cold, have aching joints, or feel tired, toxic, and like you've eaten too much of the wrong type of food.

### THE EVERGREEN BATH FOR COLDS AND COUGHS

1. Run water as hot as you can stand it into the tub. When it is almost full, add 6 drops each of pine, eucalyptus, and cypress essence. The water can be even hotter, if you fill the tub only half full, making it a kind of sitz bath.
2. Sit with your knees up and your head between them, inhaling the restorative essences. As the water cools, slosh it all over your body.
3. Get out, dry vigorously, and wrap yourself in a warm towel for a moment. Then rub your body with one of the following forest-scented oils mixed in 4 ounces of carrier oil:

    I. 2 drops of eucalyptus, 3 drops of lavender, and 2 drops of thyme
    II. 3 drops of pine, 2 drops of lemon, and 2 drops of sage
    III. 2 drops of cypress, 3 drops of geranium, and 2 drops of rosemary

### THE CLEANSING SALT BATH

This bath cleanses the system. Salt draws poisons out of the body, and sea salt contains valuable minerals that reinforce your immune system.

1. Throw two handfuls of sea salt (available in health food stores) in a tub of warm water. Mix it well with your hands and submerge yourself for ten minutes.
2. Get out, dry well, and use one of the following massage oil recipes mixed in 4 ounces of carrier oil:

    I. 2 drops of basil, 3 drops of geranium, and 3 drops of lavender
    II. 3 drops of juniper, 2 drops of sandalwood, and 3 drops of lavender
    III. 2 drops of bay, 2 drops of patchouli, and 3 drops of eucalyptus

### BATH FOR ACHES AND PAINS

Most of us have aches and pains at one time or another. Soaking in warm water is a time-honored remedy for any form of charley-horse, rheumatism, the achiness from a flu or cold, or tense and tired joints and bones.

1. Run water that is quite hot into the tub, and don't add the aromatics until the bath is almost full. Use one of the following essential-oil formulas:

   I. 4 drops of rosemary, 3 drops of chamomile, and 2 drops of thyme
   II. 4 drops of cypress, 3 drops of lavender, and 2 drops of geranium
   III. 4 drops of eucalyptus, 3 drops of pine, and 2 drops of niaouli

Dried herbs can also be added in a cheesecloth bag or in a strong tea (half a cup of herbs to 2 cups of boiling water). Try:

   I. Rosemary with lavender
   II. Sage with dried lemon peel
   III. Thyme with chamomile

Rosemary is a strong herb, but excellent for rheumatic conditions. It can be used alone, but in a not-too-concentrated solution of 2 tablespoons of herb to 1 cup of boiling water poured into a tub of water.

2. Get out and dry well. Then massage the entire body, concentrating on any aching areas with the following mixture in 4 ounces of carrier oil:

   I. 3 drops of rosemary, 2 drops of thyme, and 2 drops of lavender
   II. 3 drops of eucalyptus, 2 drops of cypress, and 2 drops of lavender
   III. 3 drops of pine, 2 drops of niaouli, and 2 drops of chamomile

## THE AROMATIC SHOWER

In our modern era of speed and convenience, showering has overtaken tubbing as the bath of choice. If you prefer a shower, you can still obtain the benefits of aromatics. Try rubbing yourself first with a little ready-made bath oil containing stimulating or relaxing essences, diluted half and half with water. Avoid the genital area, which is easily irritated. The lovely smell cascading off your body as the water rains down from above will benefit your nervous system, and some of the essences should be absorbed by your skin, making it smoother. If you do have a tub, though, try an herbal or essential-oil soak at least twice a week, using the shower before.

You can also stop up the drain while showering and sprinkle in the aromatics as the water collects. Your feet will benefit from this fragrant soak, and the aroma will ascend upward, delighting your brain.

## ___ THERAPEUTIC FOOT BATHS _____

As you already know from the other chapters, the feet communicate with the rest of the body. A foot massage, combined with an herbal or essence soak, will revive your entire system after a demanding day on your feet or night of dancing. You can soak your feet while you read, sew, knit, or write letters, adding a health-restoring activity to your leisure time.

1. Use a basin or dishpan big enough to hold your feet when they're stretched out flat, and deep enough so the water can cover your ankles. Fill it with warm water. Depending upon how you feel, choose one of the herb or essential-oil recipes recommended for the baths.
2. Before putting your feet in the water, sit in a comfortable chair and bring one foot over your knee so that you can give it a preliminary massage. Use the foot chart on page 93 to guide you, and work on each foot for about two minutes, pressing, rubbing, and pulling on each toe. Now put your feet in the basin and soak for ten minutes or more.
3. Take one foot out at a time and dry it, then rub with a massage oil of your choice. You may be surprised to find that by reviving your feet you've revived your entire body; you will feel uplifted and ready to walk another ten miles.

## ___ APPLYING AFTER-BATH MASSAGE OILS _____

After bathing, your skin is especially receptive to the wonder-working essences. A good massage oil should be quickly absorbed into the skin, and you should be able to dress within five minutes after application. If you have several different massage oils on hand, you can wake up in the morning and choose the one that suits your needs for the day. Will you need fortifying stimulation, or relaxing and calming? Are your sinuses bothering you? Do you feel achy? In the evening you can ask yourself if you are in a romantic mood, or if you want to drift off into a dreamless sleep. Then select the appropriate combination of essences.

Spread on the oils as you would any body lotion, with the following extra therapeutic movements:

1. Pour a teaspoon of oil into the center of your palm. Rub your hands together, then apply to the breasts and buttocks with a circular motion.

2. With a tiny amount of additional oil, rub your solar plexus counterclockwise six times. Then stroke the oil upward on your stomach with both hands.

3. Pour another teaspoon of oil into your palms, rub your hands together, and stroke up each arm, moving from hand to shoulder. (All moves on the limbs should be in the direction toward the heart to help circulation and lymph flow.) Grasp the arm as you slide up it with your fingers for a deeper effect.

4. Using another teaspoon of oil, work upward on your legs, stroking as deeply as possible. Move from the ankle to the top of the thigh, working with both hands, one leg at a time.

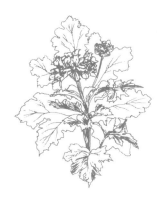

# VII

# SCENTUAL BEAUTY

Beauty *is* in the eye of the beholder, and the most important beholder is *you.* If you think you look wonderful, chances are the rest of the world will think so too. This happens because other people are most often attracted to the positive attitudes we project about our appearance. A radiant self-confidence about the way you look reflects not only the knowledge and concern you put into your style and grooming, but the vitality that comes from caring about your health. We all know men and women who by no means fulfill our idealized concepts of physical beauty, but whose intense energy and obvious sense of physical and mental well-being makes them irresistible.

## THE REVEALING FIRST STEP

The first step to self-confident attractiveness is to give your entire body a scrutinizing once-over in a well-lighted mirror; a magnified hand mirror will help you examine your face. This takes some courage, as almost no one will like everything he or she sees. Many of the problems you observe are bound to be connected to the basic condition of your skin and hair. Does your face shine with a robust glow, or is it lifeless, gray-colored, coarse in texture, or blemished? What about the skin on your body? Is it smooth, resilient, and toned, or is it flabby and lumpy, with unattractive bulges of cellulite? Does your hair shine with life and have a natural spring, or is it thin and lifeless? Questions of style can be handled by fashion consultants, makeup artists, and hair salons, but Aromatherapy's therapeutic touch techniques, plus the fragrant benefits of essential oils, combine to improve the basic slate you ask these experts to work upon. The massage and bathing systems described in previous chapters, plus the health and beauty regimens to follow, should make your face and figure a pleasure to have and behold.

Before you investigate the art of scentual beauty, identify your problems, and set some practical goals and a time frame in which to meet them. You may want smoother, more glowing skin in one month, or less cellulite on your thighs in two; you may expect an improvement in the condition of your hair and nails in six weeks. Don't reach for the sky, but try for gradual, definite changes. Decide what improvements you hope to make, which problem-solving practices to incorporate into your daily and weekly beauty routines, and then follow them diligently. You will find your beauty goals are within reach.

## YOUR BIRTHDAY SUIT

You come into the world clad in one outfit you can never completely change—your skin. This attractive wrapper is your basic wardrobe for life, and it merits serious attention. Instead, it often clings to us, neglected and unappreciated, showing the sad effects of environmental wear and tear and lack of care.

It may surprise you to learn that your skin is an important and active organ—like the liver or the heart. This organ weighs about seven pounds and measures up to eighteen square feet; just one square inch of it contains a yard of blood vessels, twenty-five nerve endings, one hundred sweat glands, and over three million cells.

The skin exists mainly to protect. It functions as a living, breathing suit of armor that keeps our vital systems and organs safely inside, and environmental invaders outside. The biological guardian also eliminates wastes, manufactures vitamins, and with its thousands of sensory nerve endings warns of danger and alerts us to pleasurable stimuli. If that isn't enough, the skin is responsible for growing hair and regulating the body's temperature. It can absorb both harmful and beneficial substances into its deepest layers, which is why it is so positively affected by the therapeutic essential oils.

There are three main layers of skin: The subcutaneous, or bottom layer, contains muscle and fatty tissue that give your skin a toned and firm appearance. The dermis is where the sensory nerves, blood vessels, lymph vessels, hair follicles, and the sebaceous and sweat glands attached to them reside. (See Diagram 11.) The epidermis or top layer is the layer we see, and is composed of flat, essentially dead cells, also known as the *stratum corneum*. Cells manufactured at the dermal level travel up to the outer layer, or epidermis—a process that is very important to the health and appearance of your skin. As the cells reach the skin's surface they form a covering, one over the other, rather like a shingled roof. There they lose their nuclei and die; eventually they are shed and new cells from below replace them. The more rapidly the dead cells on the epidermis are replaced by new ones from below, the smoother your skin looks. Lifeless cells that cling to the surface

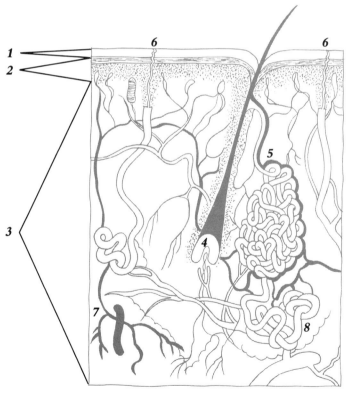

1. Stratum Corneum
2. Epidermis
3. Dermis
4. Hair bulb and shaft
5. Sweat gland
6. Apocrine (scent) gland
7. Nerves
8. Lymph vessels and arteries

*SKIN CHART*
*Diagram 11*

create a tired-looking skin, which makes you look tired too. If the outer layer of cells does not lie smoothly, due to lack of water or nutrients, it does not refract the light, and your skin appears dry and older.

## ___ THE REAL SECRET OF BEAUTIFUL SKIN ___

Cosmetics can improve lackluster skin, but no cosmetic can supply the beauty or lasting benefits of inner health. Without the right nutrition and exercise, it is almost impossible to have truly attractive skin. I say *almost*, because we all know the individual with a slim figure and flawless complexion who eats only junk food, and whose exercise regimen consists of marathon television watching. Of course, these lucky souls are usually fourteen, or possess an incredible gene bank. Inheritance is a key factor in how we look and how we age. Because your fair-skinned mother was wrinkled at sixty, however, does not necessarily mean you have to be. I believe in taking note of the weaknesses you are likely to inherit—in both your appearance and your health—and heading them off at the pass!

The skin is so affected by your health and state of mind that it is a virtual mirror of your mental and physical condition. A professional Aromatherapist, as we have already discussed, makes an initial diagnosis of the client's health by examining the skin. Its color, texture, and resiliency reveal what the organs, nerves, and circulatory system are up to. If your skin lacks color, luster, and tone, the first step to improving it is to take a good look at your life-style, diet, and mental attitude. A diet that is high in fats, sugar, and refined foods and low in natural grains, raw fruits, and vegetables, and a life-style that includes smoking and drinking, lack of exercise, plus tension, fear, or anger, add up to dull, blemished, or prematurely aging skin.

Though nothing you can do to your skin on the outside will totally compensate for poor inner maintenance, the care you give your complexion can definitely improve its overall appearance. My Aromatherapy skin maintenance program will provide even better results if you also make positive changes in your health habits. The program offers some excellent techniques to correct and maintain your skin's condition. These include cleansing, balancing, stimulating, hydrating, and nourishing. These procedures enhance the top layer of the skin by stimulating cell production in its deepest layers, and by smoothing and disinfecting the surface with essential oils. Many commercial cosmetic products promise to accomplish the same result, but tend to work only on the surface of the skin, and achieve only temporary benefits if they achieve anything at all. Moreover, many are loaded with synthetic scents and materials that are not only ineffective, but can damage some sensitive skins. For this reason, I have suggested certain types of products and have given recipes for skin-care solutions you can make yourself.

## ___ SCENTUAL CLEANSING _____

Before you can treat the skin it must be clean. The environment (especially in cities) and the skin itself produce impurities that have to be removed before the skin can benefit from ingredients that nourish, smooth, and soothe. Hundreds of minute oil sacs, or sebaceous glands, just beneath the surface of the face push oil up through the same follicle tubes that grow fine facial hairs. The residue of the skin-manufacturing process is also thrown out with the oil—a gunky mixture called *sebum.* When too much sebum is produced (which can be caused by hormones, hot weather, diet, and tension), it plugs up the pores. A clogged pore is unreceptive to treatment. Moreover, this sebum deposit can turn black and become a *blackhead*—a minor skin blemish, not caused by dirt from the outside, as many believe, but by the skin itself. A pimple occurs when an infection develops in a follicle overloaded with impurities and bacteria.

If you want to avoid unsightly blemishes, then, and have a skin that glows with oxygen-rich vitality, you must get it scrupulously clean. *How* you clean is very important, because you must get the pore-stopping impurities *out* as well as *off.* Strong soaps and vigorous scrubbing will cleanse thoroughly, but they will also strip your skin of its precious acid mantle. This acidity, which maintains the pH of the skin, wards off bacteria and helps keep it smooth. Because regular soap is very alkaline, it destroys the acidity, making your skin feel taut and dry.

Getting your skin clean and restoring its acid mantle is a two-step process: first you cream and wash, then you balance, or tone. This two-part technique works equally well for dry and oily skin, because you can vary the products and procedures according to your needs. (See the section "Aromatherapy Skin Maintenance Program" on page 156.) There are, however, several basic rules to observe for cleansing any type of skin:

1. *Never use your hands.* The warmth and magnetism of your hands can actually push the dirt and impurities back into the pores. Use a cotton ball, saturated with a cream cleanser, for each section of your face: forehead, cheeks, nose, chin, and throat.

2. *Wash with a thick, white washcloth.* After you apply your cleanser with cotton, wash it off with warm water and a thick, white terry washcloth, which will stimulate your skin with mild friction. You can always judge the cleanliness of a white washcloth. I recommend buying seven—one for each day of the week.

3. *Cleanse twice a day.* You do it for your teeth, why not for your face, which is even more visible? Many women clean their faces only at night to remove makeup, but wouldn't dream of cleansing in the morning before they apply makeup. As a result, they create a bacteria-loaded occlusion of oil, powder, and coloring agents over sebum and dead skin scales. The skin is just as in need of cleansing after a night's sleep as it is after a day in the polluted city. At night your skin throws off body toxins and produces new cells, which push away the old—a good reason, by the way, to change your sheets and pillowcases at least twice a week. A microscope would show you a lively population of dead skin and microscopic creatures on the bedclothes you've been sleeping on for a couple of days.

## ____ *SCENTUAL BALANCING* ____

A mild freshener, or a slightly stronger toner, can help restore the acid mantle of your skin after cleansing. Both the freshener and the toner contain acids and salts that refurbish the skin's pH, or its natural chemical balance. No matter how oily your skin, I don't believe you should use a strong, alcohol-based astringent. It will strip your skin of its protective mantle, and encourage the overactive oil glands to produce more oil to compensate for the alcohol's drying action.

You can buy a freshener or toner (be sure it is not alcohol-based), or you can make your own. The following mixtures will keep for at least a month.

*Dry Skin Freshener #1*

Boil 1 pint of water and steep four chamomile tea bags (or 2 heaping teaspoons of chamomile) in it for one minute. Add 6 drops of a citrus-type essence, like lemon, tangerine, or orange, when cool. Shake well in a tightly covered bottle before using.

*Dry Skin Freshener #2*

Boil 1 pint of water and steep four rosehip tea bags for one minute in it. Add 6 drops of lavender essence when cool. Shake in a tightly covered bottle before using.

*Oily Skin Toner #1*

Boil 1 pint of water and steep two chamomile and two comfrey root tea bags in it (or 2 heaping teaspoons of each of the herbs). Add 6 drops of juniper essence when cool. Shake well in a tightly covered bottle before using.

*Oily Skin Toner #2*

Boil 1 pint of water with two lemongrass and two ginseng tea bags (or 2 heaping teaspoons each of the lemongrass and pure ginseng powder) and add 6 drops of sage essence. Shake well.

All fresheners and toners should be applied with cotton squares or balls. Work them over the face, using little circles, then blot dry with a facial tissue. *Do not rub* a tissue over your face, no matter how soft; paper products contain small wooden fibers that can rough up the surface of your skin.

____ *SCENTUAL MOISTURIZING* _____

Probably the most commonly used—and misused—cosmetic on the market today is the moisturizer. The basic concept of the moisturizer is sound: it prevents the skin from losing water by sealing it in with an oil and water emulsion. However, a moisturizer should not obstruct the skin's ability to take in nutrients, eliminate debris, and breathe. Unfortunately, many of them do just that.

What we call "dry skin" is not so much a skin that has lost its water supply as it is a skin whose scaly top layer has been roughed up. If the way these dead cells are arranged—neatly tucked into one another—is disturbed, the skin looks and feels very dry. An alkaline soap, deficient diet, or harsh environmental factors can disturb the top layer. A good moisturizer should smooth out the cells, while it locks water into them. The trick is to find a product with natural, active moisturizing ingredients, including essential oils, and *without* mineral oil. Mineral oil is made from petroleum and is incompatible with the fats in human skin. It lies like a film over the skin, forming a barrier, so that nothing can get in or out. Skin needs to breathe. Mineral oil is also known to leach fat-soluble vitamins out of the body, which is why most doctors have stopped prescribing it as a laxative. These vitamins, A, D, and E, are vital to your skin's state of health.

After you clean and tone your face, leaving the skin just a bit damp, apply a moisturizer that does not contain mineral oil. Put about a quarter of a teaspoon of moisturizer into the palm of one hand, then spread it gently over your face and neck with the other. If the moisturizer is a liquid, pour just a few drops into the palm of your hand. If it is more solid and packaged in a jar, do not dip your fingers into the jar. Instead use a small scoop, like a little wooden mustard spoon, to remove the cream. Every time you put your fingers in a jar you introduce a colony of bacteria into it. Even if your product is protected by preservatives, some of these germs may survive, and sponsor an eye infection or a skin breakout. While I'm on the subject of germs, always wash your hands before you touch your face. If you could see the microbes you pick up in just a few hours of average activity, you would never touch your face again without scrubbing your hands.

## SCENTUAL NOURISHING

Your face is fed much more by the nutrients you consume in your diet than by any substance you can apply to your skin. However, both the internal and external approaches work synergistically, especially in a clean environment. The cleaner your skin is, the better it can utilize nutrients.

Starting with the inside, your skin needs vitamins and minerals, plus living enzymes, obtained only from raw food. A number of vitamins are important to the skin. Vitamins A and D work together to heal the skin's external and internal layers. Vitamin E keeps fats from turning into free radicals, which can cause cell abnormality on the inside, and heals and brings oxygen to the cells on the outside. Vitamin C promotes capillary strength and helps maintain collagen, the protein that keeps your skin firm and resilient. (Cigarette smoking, by the way, destroys the body's supply of vitamin C, one of the reasons heavy smokers develop deeper facial lines than nonsmokers.) The B vitamins feed the nerves and muscles. The mineral zinc keeps the skin elastic, and sulfur strengthens the skin, hair, and nails. Selenium works like vitamin E to prevent oxidation and aging, and silicon makes the hair shiny and the skin firm. Iodine strengthens both hair and nails. One of the reasons Japanese women have such strong, beautiful hair is because their diet includes iodine-rich seaweed. Calcium and magnesium work to utilize the other nutrients. Any good book on nutrition will tell you which natural foods contain the skin-essential vitamins and minerals; dietary supplements can be taken as well.

The face can also be nourished from the outside. Some creams, oils, and lotions are better than others and provide visible, long-lasting effects. Again, stay away from any product containing mineral oil, and look for those that emphasize natural ingredients, vitamins, and essential oils. It is unnecessary to nourish your skin with heavy, greasy creams; these block your pores at night, when your skin should shed impurities and dead cells and breathe. Try to find a formulation rich enough to lubricate your skin, but which doesn't leave a greasy film. A light nourishing face oil of essential oils in a vegetable oil base can be made at home. Try the following combinations:

*Nourishing Oil for Dry and/or Mature Skin*
Combine one-half ounce of avocado oil and one-half ounce of wheat germ oil with 3 ounces of vegetable oil, such as almond, soy, or sesame. Then add:

   6 drops of lavender
   3 drops of geranium (or rose if you can afford it)

3 drops of sandalwood
800 units of vitamin E (squeeze a vitamin capsule into the oil)

Combine all ingredients and shake well. Pour one-half teaspoon of the mixture into the palm of one hand, and apply over face and neck with the other.

*Nourishing Oil for Oily Skin*
In 3 ounces of light vegetable oil, such as safflower or sunflower, add:

6 drops of chamomile
4 drops of sage
4 drops of basil
800 units of vitamin E

Mix and apply as above.

Cleansing, balancing, moisturizing, and nourishing must be done daily. You can further enhance the quality of your skin by stimulating and hydrating it. These procedures are an essential part of skin care, though they need not be done on a daily basis.

## SCENTUAL STIMULATING

Good blood circulation is the key to healthy, attractive skin. The circulatory system works from within to promote delivery of oxygen and nutrients to the skin (as well as to other organs) and to remove waste products. A lively flow of blood and lymph also stimulates cell turnover, and tones muscles and nerves. Most of this circulatory activity occurs in the skin's second layer, the dermis. There are four effective ways to increase circulation to the facial and body skin: (1) exercise that is vigorous enough to make you sweat, (2) massage, (3) inversion, and (4) masks and wraps with herbs and essential oils.

*Exercise*
Without exercise, an all-important circulation booster, the effectiveness of every other routine you pursue for health and beauty is weakened. Choose

a method of exercise and do it consistently. Make sure you choose one that increases your heart rate and makes you perspire, giving your face a visible glow. Sweating is an important cleansing process for the entire body, as well as for the skin.

*Massage*

The massage movements explained in Chapters III and IV, and the self-massage you do in your aroma bath, are designed to stimulate the circulatory and nervous systems as well as the skin. In addition, I recommend a special facial massage technique called *tapping*. (See Illustration VII–1.) Whenever you apply face oils, moisturizers, or nourishing creams, tap briskly with the fingertips of both hands, concentrating on the areas that tend to line and crease, such as the forehead, around the mouth, and on the chin line. Tap

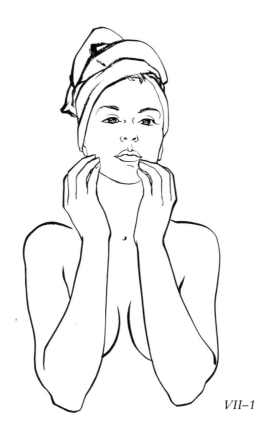

VII–1

each area ten times. This makes the cells "greedier" for the treatment you apply and tones facial muscles.

Pressures on key points on the face stimulate major organs and are also highly beneficial for the skin. (Consult the face chart, Diagram 12, for the important point locations.) Don't forget that the skin is an eliminatory organ. Activating other eliminatory organs, like the kidneys and colon, with therapeutic pressures can help clear the skin, since these other organs can rid the

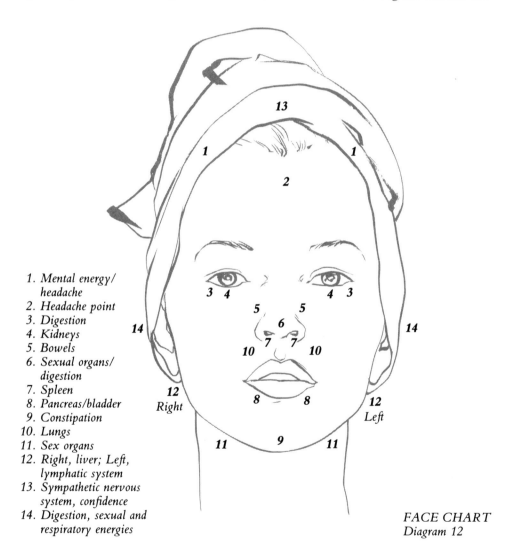

1. Mental energy/
   headache
2. Headache point
3. Digestion
4. Kidneys
5. Bowels
6. Sexual organs/
   digestion
7. Spleen
8. Pancreas/bladder
9. Constipation
10. Lungs
11. Sex organs
12. Right, liver; Left,
    lymphatic system
13. Sympathetic nervous
    system, confidence
14. Digestion, sexual and
    respiratory energies

FACE CHART
Diagram 12

body of toxins that might otherwise have to pass through the skin, causing cloudiness and blemishes. Pressures are best done after you clean your face and sparingly apply a facial massage oil. Use the second and third fingers of both hands simultaneously on both sides of the face on corresponding points. Hold each pressure for a count of ten. The pressures will only take about two minutes, and will make you feel and look better for hours.

### Inversion

Putting your feet over your head is a relaxed yet efficient way to send healing, nourishing blood into your face and to tone your colon at the same time. The colon is shaped like an upside-down U; the part that runs horizontally across the upper abdomen begins to droop in the middle as we get older. The best way to invert yourself is to lie on a slant board, which keeps your body in a straight line, feet higher than head. The colon will fall up into place, allowing it to work better, at least while you are inverted.

As you lie with your feet up, your face and head will be fed by your circulatory system, making your eyes brighter and your brain clearer. Twenty minutes on a slant board is worth forty-five of lying flat in terms of revitalization. The slant board can be a life saver if you're tired and your rest time is limited. Try it after work or a day of hectic shopping, or as an antidote to a tiring night. You can multiply its benefits by cleansing your face, applying a stimulating herbed mask, and placing cotton squares dipped in cool chamomile tea over your eyes.

Department stores and athletic supply stores carry slant boards (which can also be used for tummy-flattening sit-ups), or you can make your own, using a two foot wide by six foot long board. The end where your head will rest should be on the floor, and the foot end should be propped up fifteen inches. The board you buy will be padded, but if you're using a homemade version you should soften it with a folded blanket. In a pinch you can substitute a full-sized ironing board with the legs folded, and prop it up on a low chair or hassock. I have given myself a much-needed energy boost on many a hotel ironing board. Just call room service and tell them your suit is wrinkled and you want to iron it, then get set for a refreshing beauty break.

### Masks and Wraps

An essential part of the stimulating process for facial skin is a mask, which also cleanses. You can actually use a nondrying mask as your morning cleanser. (See my suggestions in the section "Aromatherapy Skin Maintenance Program" on page 156 for masks for normal, dry, and oily skins.) Let the mask sit for about five minutes while you make the bed or set out your clothes for the day, then rinse it off with warm water.

Clay is the queen of masks; like the essential oils, it is a completely natural, skin-friendly substance, which contains nourishing minerals and other active, cleansing substances. Clay also has polarity properties; its negative electric charge acts as a magnet to toxins, which have a positive charge, pulling them into it. Clay is also mildly radioactive; for this reason, European spas have utilized it for centuries to heal arthritis and rheumatism.

The fantastically absorbent action of clay makes it a good body powder, and even a deodorant, as well as a stimulating and cleansing mask. You can buy natural clay (sometimes called "Fuller's Earth") in some pharmacies and most health food stores. To make a simple mask, put 2 tablespoons of clay in a wooden, glass, or ceramic bowl and add 2 teaspoons of water. Let the mixture thicken and then spread it over your face, avoiding the eye area. To get the full benefit of this clay pack, leave it on for twenty minutes while its nourishing and cleansing minerals—silica, iron, calcium, magnesium, and zinc—feed your face and sabotage impurities. Rinse with warm water, and pat your face dry.

Clay is a fierce enemy of pimples and boils, because it draws out their poisons and "cools" the infected area. Just be sure to clean the territory the clay will cover first, so it can work in the deepest possible way on the problem. Because clay is so active, it can be a little drying; fine or dry skins should be treated with it only once a week, and oily skins twice.

## SCENTUAL HYDRATING

The skin needs water to maintain its health and smooth texture. There are a number of ways to "water" your facial skin—both from the inside and outside. First, you must drink enough pure, spring water to cleanse your body and moisten your skin. You get a certain amount of water from fruits, vegetables, and their juices and from herbal teas and other beverages. At least twice a day, however, you should drink eight ounces of water.

You can moisturize your face from the outside by rinsing off cleansers and masks with warm water. Close your eyes, and let the spray from your shower rain down on your face.

Steaming is an aromatic way to hydrate your skin. When steam is combined with herbs and/or essences, it can cleanse your pores and stimulate at the same time. You can buy a facial steamer, or put your hot infusion in a bowl. Cover your head with a towel, and let your thirsty skin inhale the fragrant steam. (See Illustration VII–2.) Try the following steaming combinations.

### Dried-Herb Infusion Steam

*For Dry to Normal Skin.* Simmer 1 ounce of chamomile, 2 ounces of lemongrass, and 1 ounce of peppermint in a quart of boiling water for ten minutes. Pour into bowl. When mixture is slightly cooled, but still steaming, put a towel over your head, close your eyes, and allow the steam to work for five minutes.

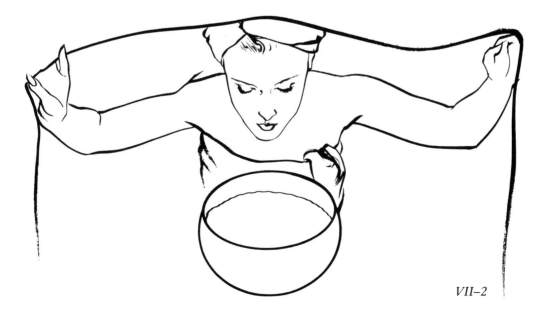

*VII–2*

*For Oily Skin.* Follow the above instructions, but simmer 1 ounce of comfrey root, 1 ounce of rosemary, and 1 ounce of basil in a quart of boiling water.

### Essential-Oil Steam

*For Dry to Normal, and Mature Skin.* Heat a quart of water to the boiling point. Let it cool slightly and add 4 drops of geranium, 4 drops of lavender, and 2 drops of patchouli. Quickly cover your head and the bowl with a towel, so the essences will not evaporate. Steam for five minutes.

*For Oily Skin.* Follow the above instructions, but add 4 drops of lemon essence, 4 drops of cypress, and 6 drops of juniper to the water.

After steaming the skin should be balanced with a toner or freshener, and a light moisturizer should be applied.

Air travel is deadly drying. Carry a small aerosol can of mineral water, available in most pharmacies and in some department stores, and spray your face every hour or so during the flight. Step up your beverage intake while aloft, but don't drink any alcohol. Alcohol is very dehydrating, and its damaging effect on the skin is multiplied in high altitudes.

## ____AROMATHERAPY SKIN MAINTENANCE PROGRAM____

Effective skin care demands a basic morning and night routine, which you must practice without fail. Below is my cleansing, balancing, stimulating, moisturizing, and nourishing program for dry and/or normal and oily skin. To these routines you may want to add the additional stimulating benefits of steaming, inversion, and massage.

### FOR DRY AND/OR NORMAL SKIN

#### Morning Maintenance

1. Apply moisturizing mask (nondrying cream type). Allow five minutes to set and perform cleansing, stimulating action.
2. Wash off mask, using a thick terry washcloth and warm, not hot, water.
3. Soak cotton square in mild face freshener (see recipes under "Scentual

Balancing," page 146). Wipe over face. Pat dry (don't rub) with facial tissue.

4. Pour small amount of face oil (see recipes under "Scentual Nourishing," page 148) in palm of hand. Sweep in upward motion over face and neck (except for nose). Tap into skin on forehead, around the mouth, jawline, under eyes and neck. Allow oil to penetrate the skin for at least half an hour.
5. Apply moisturizer before makeup base.

### Night Maintenance

1. Remove dirt and/or makeup with cream- or milk-type cleanser on a separate cotton ball for each section of the face. Apply with upward and outward motions. Work gently on eyelid area. If you prefer to remove your mascara with a commercial remover, this is the time to do that.
2. Wash off cleanser with warm, not hot, water, using a thick terry washcloth. Wash off mascara with a cream-type cleansing bar (this is not actually soap, but a nonalkaline cleanser) if you prefer this method of removal.
3. Soak cotton square with freshener and wipe over entire face and neck. Pat dry with a tissue.
4. Apply about a quarter of a teaspoon of nourishing cream or oil. Use a scoop if it is a cream, or pour the oil into your hand. Dot over face and smooth in. Tap areas that line, like forehead, the area under eyes, around the mouth, chin and neck.

If your skin becomes more oily, follow the program instructions for oily skin below. Return to this routine when your skin becomes dry again.

### FOR OILY SKIN

#### Morning Maintenance

1. Apply a stimulating mask. This could be a cream-type product with essences such as rosemary, thyme, geranium, or juniper. Twice a week use pure clay as a mask. Leave mask on long enough to dry and stimulate, about ten minutes.
2. Wash mask off with a thick terry washcloth and warm water.

3. Apply a toner (somewhat stronger and more stimulating than a freshener, but should not contain alcohol; see recipes under "Scentual Balancing," page 146) with a cotton square. Pat dry (don't rub) with a facial tissue.

4. Apply a light moisturizer, tapping it into areas that line, like the forehead, under-eye area, jawline, and around the mouth.

### Night Maintenance

1. Remove dirt and/or makeup with milk-type cleanser. Use a cotton ball for each section of the face, wiping upward and outward. Move gently over eyelid area. If you remove mascara with a commercial product, do it now.

2. Wash off cleanser with a thick terry washcloth, using a cream-type bar (not an alkaline soap) and warm water. Rinse well. Remove mascara at the same time, if you prefer to wash it off.

3. Soak cotton square with toner and wipe over entire face and neck. Pat dry with a tissue.

4. Apply a face oil for oily skin (see recipes under "Scentual Nourishing," page 148). Pour about a quarter of a teaspoon of oil into the palm and sweep into the face with the other hand. Tap into areas that line with both hands.

## _____ SCENTUAL HAND CARE _____

Your hands communicate who you are and what you think. You don't have to be born with attractive hands; you can develop them. What you *do* with your hands affects their appearance in important ways. Practicing Aromatherapy massage actually improves the way hands look and increases their expressive abilities. Massage gives the muscles and tendons of the hands important exercise. Also, the fact that you are touching in a loving as well as therapeutic manner seems to give your hands new meaning; you will feel their positive power as never before. The essential oils, too, renew the skin of your hands and build the health of your nails. My own hands have become younger every year that I have practiced Aromatherapy; so will yours.

Exercises, self-massage, and consistent hand care will make your hands look younger and stronger, and will help you give yourself and others a more beneficial massage.

### BEAUTIFUL HAND EXERCISES

#### 1. Fingertip Push

Place your hands in the prayer position, palm to palm. Push the tips of your fingers together, opening the heels of your hands. Push as hard as you can for a count of ten. Relax and push again. Repeat six times. The fingertip push strengthens your lower arm and wrist, as well as your hands.

#### 2. Ball Squeeze

Buy two small rubber balls at the dime store. Keep them handy to squeeze while you wait for your tub to run or your mask to dry. You can also pick them up while watching television or talking on the phone. (You may want to use a foam rubber "gripper" which is found in the weight-lifting department of an athletic supply store instead.) Squeeze with a ball in each hand as hard and long as you can.

#### 3. Invisible Keys

Place your fingers on a table or desk and pretend you are playing a sonata on an invisible keyboard. Play with your fingers curved, creating your masterwork, while you make your fingers more flexible and sensitive.

### HAND SOAK AND STROKE

Soaking and massaging your hands and nails with an essence-rich oil will definitely improve their look and feel. As I suggested in Chapter VI in the aroma bath, wash your hands with mild soap and rinse well before you soak them. This treatment is especially beneficial for rough, dry hands.

Fill a 2-quart bowl with 1 quart of warm (not hot) water. Pour in 1 cup of strong chamomile tea (made with 2 heaping teaspoons of chamomile or two tea bags). Add 6 drops of lavender and 6 drops of geranium essence. Immerse your hands in the solution for ten minutes. You can use it again to soak your feet, or pour it into your bathwater after your extemities have enjoyed it.

Pat your hands dry and smooth in the following hand oil:

In 2 ounces of sesame oil and 1 ounce each of almond and avocado oil, mix:

6 drops of lavender
6 drops of chamomile
6 drops of sandalwood
800 units of vitamin E, squeezed from a capsule.

Mix by gently shaking the bottle.

Pour one-half teaspoon of this fragrant, therapeutic oil into the palm of one hand, stroking it in with a pulling motion from wrist to fingers. Then massage each finger and end by rubbing each nail to bring healing, stimulating blood into the fingertips. This will promote nail strength and growth. Pour another half teaspoon of oil into the other hand, and massage it, using the same technique.

Both the oil and the massage technique can be used on your feet.

## ___WRAPS AND OILS FOR CELLULITE___

Cellulite is a lumpy, dimpled fat deposit that clings maddeningly to the outer thighs, hips, and buttocks, and sometimes to the upper arms. Quite different from ordinary fat, cellulite is a repository for extra water and toxic waste, which is why it is so hard to banish. European spas and Aromatherapists treat this unattractive "orange-peel skin" and other fatty deposits with special diets, massage, and wraps with herbal infusions and essences, which draw the toxins out and encourage the elimination of water.

Before you wrap, massage the fatty area with firm, upward strokes, using the essential-oil mixtures suggested below:

*Cellulite Massage Oil #1*
To 4 ounces of a light vegetable oil, like safflower or sunflower, add:

6 drops of lavender
6 drops of juniper
10 drops of rosemary

Shake well.

### *Cellulite Massage Oil #2*
To 4 ounces of oil add:

6 drops of geranium
6 drops of sage
10 drops of cypress

Shake well.

You are now ready to wrap the area in a soaking solution of herbal infusions. You will need a large roll of wide surgical gauze, and a roll of plastic wrap. Dip the gauze in one of the solutions below, then wrap the area around several times in the wet gauze. Cover that with the plastic covering.

### *Cellulite Wrap Formula #1*
Simmer the following herbs in 1 quart of water for ten minutes. Cool and strain.

1 ounce of dried rosemary
1 ounce of dried sage
1 ounce of chamomile

### *Cellulite Wrap Formula #2*
Simmer in 1 quart of water. Cool and strain.

1 ounce of thyme
1 ounce of sage
2 large strips of seaweed (Kombu or Nori)

Lie down for twenty minutes, and let the herbs and essences stimulate the tissues, helping them to eliminate water and poisons. Unwrap and throw all the wrappings away (they contain waste, and should not be reused). Repeat this process twice a week. This massage/wrap method diminishes fatty tissue, especially when combined with the right diet, which will be described in Chapter VIII, and the dry brush massage, which was described in Chapter VI.

## SCENTUAL HAIR CARE

The hair, like the skin, reflects your state of mental and physical health. Worry, illness, or poor nutrition thin and dull the hair, making it unmanageable. The same philosophy that applies to the skin also applies to the hair: hair needs to be nourished both from the inside and outside, and the cleaner it is the better it functions.

The hair bulb, or root, is formed in the second layer of skin, the dermis. Tiny blood vessels feed the bulb the ingredients it needs to make hair from *keratin*, the same material that forms your nails. Keratin is made up of proteins, and without sufficient protein in the diet our hair and nails will not be healthy and strong. However, you can have beautiful hair without eating large quantities of fatty or cholesterol-laden animal proteins, like steaks, eggs, and dairy products. You can find amino acids, the hair protein builders, in a balanced vegetarian diet, which will be discussed in Chapter VIII.

The scalp is stimulated by Aromatherapy massage techniques, described in Chapters III and IV. Lying on the slant board also promotes hair growth, since it sends blood into the head. Another way to encourage the circulatory system to feed the hair is to bend over and massage your scalp with your fingers, *moving* the scalp, instead of sliding over the hair. Then put one drop of bay essence in your palm and rub it over the bristles of a natural-bristle hairbrush. Bend over and brush from the scalp out to the ends of the hair. The bay essence, a prime ingredient in turn-of-the-century hair tonics, will stimulate growth and leave your hair smelling crisply clean.

Shampoo your hair at least every other day with a mild nondetergent shampoo. A few drops of lavender or chamomile oil added to the shampoo increases its cleansing properties. Rinse well, then pour a pint of chamomile tea over the hair as a second rinse. The chamomile soothes the scalp and adds highlights to blond or light brown hair. Brunettes can take a tip from Indian women, who have beautiful lustrous black hair, and rinse with 6 drops of sandalwood essence in 1 pint of water. This makes dark hair strong and shiny, and gives it an enticing aroma.

### *Hair-Nail Oil Soak*

Your hair and nails will both benefit from an occasional soak in essential oils. Warm 6 ounces of sesame or soy oil and pour it into a small bowl. Add 6 drops of lavender, 6 drops of bay, and 6 drops of sandalwood. With a large wad of cotton apply the oil to your scalp, parting the hair an inch at a time, working from one side of the head to the other. Then wrap your head in a towel and soak your fingertips in the remaining oil for fifteen minutes while you watch television or listen to your favorite recording. You will have to soap your hair twice to get the oil out. Your hair should be silky and manageable when you've finished this treatment, and your cuticles and hands will be softer and smoother.

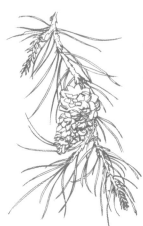

# VIII

# THE ESSENCE
# OF HEALTH

How you look and feel affect the way you choose to live your life. It is important that you think not merely about your appearance and energy level today, but also about ten years from today. Aromatherapy provides time-honored beauty and health practices that can make your present more rewarding and ensure your future well-being.

As you begin your search for the essence of health, keep in mind that your body wants to help you. Unless you are the victim of a severe genetic mistake, your body is designed to function and wants to be well. Even when we radically depart from all the norms of self-care, our body and mind struggle to pull us back to inner stability. Like any efficiently engineered machine, there is a level at which the human organism runs best, with no blips, squeaks, or vibrations. The Aromatherapy way to achieve maximum body efficiency depends on the same system that you used to care for your skin: clean, balance, stimulate, and nourish.

## _____ AROMATHERAPY BODY CLEANSING _____

You must clean the inside of your body just as you clean the outside. The body is in a constant state of mild toxemia as a result of its natural metabolic functions. It conducts a never-ending cell replacement program, renewing between three and eight hundred *billion* cells a day. On top of that, it becomes laden with debris left by food that is not properly digested and assimilated (that is, taken in by the cells). This debris, which is mildly toxic, or poisonous, is increased or decreased by the way we live and eat.

Is there anything wrong with being a little toxic? Everybody is, and, most of the time, you won't even be aware of this sludge of debris in your body. Unfortunately, while toxicity may go unnoticed on a day-to-day level, it is potentially deadly. Many health experts believe that these toxins are responsible for a host of diseases, as well as obesity and negative mental and emotional conditions. Chronic fatigue is one of toxicity's major warning signs. Fatigue commonly plagues people in "civilized" industrial countries— the chronically tired are usually the chronically polluted. Many people believe they feel tired because they have "overdone it" physically or mentally, or because they have "burnout" jobs, but if you wake up tired, having slept a good night's sleep, you are tired because you are toxic.

Your system will help you deal with toxicity if you give it half a chance. It's really very simple. First you allow your body to clean itself out through its natural elimination processes, and then you improve the quality of what you put in. Henceforth, you think more carefully about when and how you fuel your energy system.

### The Modified Fast

A fast is an excellent way to houseclean your system. Stringent fasting, with professional supervision, is the best way to cleanse, but few of us have the time, money, or even the willpower to take a foodless vacation at an expensive spa. There are also some health conditions that make hard-core fasting on water and/or juice dangerous. Hypoglycemia, or low blood sugar, is one of them. Hypoglycemics need to eat often, and stay away from sweet and refined foods, or else they immediately feel weak, faint, and extremely irritable. I come from a long line of hypoglycemics (both my mother and father had low blood sugar), and fasting for any length of time makes me feel dizzy, shaky, and decidedly unwell.

A modified twenty-four-hour fast, recommended to me by Micheline Arcier, can be a good safe start to cleansing your system. It can also put you on the road to sensible weight loss, if part of your goal is to shed extra pounds. This modified fast should not interrupt your normal life, even if you work every day in an office. Before you embark on this fast, or on any of the dietary suggestions in this chapter, however, you should check with a nutrition-oriented doctor (not always easy to find). Everybody's system is unique and has different requirements. Instead of fasting, you may need to slowly but surely improve the way you eat and incorporate other health practices into your life.

- *On rising* drink a large cup of hot water with the juice of half a lemon squeezed into it. Allow one hour before eating.
- *For breakfast* have fruit and yogurt with 1 teaspoon of honey and 1 tablespoon of wheat germ; or a bowl of whole-grain cereal, like meusli or Familia; or unsweetened granola, with honey, banana, and skim milk. If you have a blood sugar problem, skip the honey. Drink a cup of herbal tea, cereal coffee, or decaffeinated tea or coffee. If you must, have real coffee or tea. Don't use sugar, honey, or a chemical sugar substitute in any of the beverages.
- *For lunch* have a large salad of greens, raw vegetables, and sprouts, but no meat, hard cheese, or fish. You can add a small amount of cottage cheese or the *yolk* of a hard-boiled egg. Do not use any salad dressing that contains sugar, cheese, chemical preservatives, or MSG. Pure vegetable oil with cider vinegar or lemon, fresh garlic and herbs, like basil and tarragon, with a little salt substitute makes the best dressing. A slice of whole-grain bread with no, or almost no, butter can be eaten with the salad. Drink the same beverage as you did for breakfast.
- *With dinner*, or should I say *without dinner*, you begin your fast. Drink only a cup of hot water with lemon or a mild herb tea, such as chamomile or rosehip.
- *On rising*, drink only hot water with lemon.
- *For breakfast*, another cup of hot water with lemon, or a mild herb tea.
- *With lunch* you are ready to break the fast, but with cleansing still in mind. If you are not hypoglycemic, eat several sub-acid fresh fruits, such as peaches, nectarines, apples, and pears, and have a cup of herbal tea. If your sugar is unstable, have a medium-sized green salad with raw vegetables and two tablespoons of mixed, chopped, raw nuts (with no fat or salt). Eat slowly, and chew every bite until it dissolves. You should introduce food back into your system gently and in small quantities.
- *For dinner* have 6 ounces of freshly squeezed vegetable juice, such as carrot, celery, and parsley, a half hour before you eat. Then have a medium-sized

green salad with tomatoes and cucumbers, and a lemon or tomato juice dressing. Don't use oil. For the main course, have three lightly steamed vegetables, such as string beans, broccoli, and yellow squash with no butter or salt. Use dried herbs, such as basil, rosemary, or tarragon for flavoring and to aid digestion.

### Essential Elimination

*Elimination* is a concept most people are too squeamish to discuss. This all-important process is essential for good health and good looks. You should always be concerned about your elimination, as it is your body's natural way of ridding itself of toxins. If your small and large intestines and colon do not function well, you will not be well, no matter what else you do for your health. You should process and *easily* eliminate the waste products of what you eat within twenty-four hours. If it takes longer than that, if your stool is small and hard, or if you must strain to eliminate, you are probably constipated. You can test your waste transit time by eating something easy to track, like beets. If it takes several days to see a red-colored stool, you are running slow.

Poor elimination spells *autointoxication*, which means you are slowly but surely poisoning yourself. Arthritis, diverticulitis (or an inflammation of little sacs in the bowel), chronic gas, fatigue, colon cancer, and other problems are all the result of holding irritating, debilitating wastes in the body. To be healthy and full of energy, then, your elimination must be prompt and complete. To accomplish this you must eat natural, fiber-rich food, like whole grains and raw vegetables, drink at least six cups of liquid a day (or four cups of liquid and lots of juicy foods like fruit), and exercise enough to stimulate peristalsis (the contractions that push matter through the colon).

Colonics and enemas can start you off on a cleansing program without the handicap of a full colon. A colonic—a special enema that cleans the entire lower bowel—should be administered by a professional therapist, but you can give yourself an enema. Add 2 drops of lavender to the enema water and swish it around in the warm water. This soothes and cleans the colon.

Aromatherapy massage also helps stimulate elimination, since the nerve endings that connect with the colon are located along the spine. (See Diagram 4 on page 43 and its accompanying analysis in Chapter III.) Pressure points on the feet, hands, and face also work on the colon. (See Diagrams 9, 10, and 12 in Chapters IV and VII.) Essential oils such as rosemary, thyme, eucalyptus, bay, juniper, and lemongrass are excellent aids for a detoxifying massage. One effective combination would be 6 drops of eucalyptus, 4 drops of rosemary, and 2 drops of thyme in 4 ounces of carrier oil.

## AROMATHERAPY BODY BALANCING

When you are in balance you are not *too* anything—you are neither under-active nor overactive, too excited or too lethargic, too fat or too thin. That doesn't mean life is devoid of excitement; on the contrary, when your body is in balance you will have more energy for the activities and people you love. I once climbed to the top of a small mountain in the Himalayas to visit a renowned guru named Swami Rama. As we sat overlooking the magnif-icent scenery of Nepal, I told him that some of my contemporaries feared Eastern meditation because it might take away their "edge," making them unable to wage combat in the fast lane of our Western society and business world. The Swami just looked at me and smiled serenely. "Balance, every-thing must be done in balance," he said.

Your body instinctively understands the Swami's words. It strives to correct imbalances all the time; the trick you have to master is to let your body do its job. *Listen* to your body. If you really feel tired, lie down and rest. If you aren't hungry, don't eat. When you reach the point of exhaustion, stop exercising. Going beyond your limits, and defying messages from the conscious and subconscious brain, will usually get you in trouble. Pain and exhaustion are nature's way of informing you that something is wrong. Stimulating your overtired system with caffeinated drinks, relaxing with alcohol, or masking pain with drugs only briefly postpones the reckoning—illness or collapse. Find out *why* you have the headache, back pain, fatigue, or tension, and do something about it.

### Tension

Tension is an unbalanced situation for both your body and your mind and Aromatherapy massage is one of the best ways to cure it. Whether you are massaged by someone else or yourself, the therapeutic touch and essential oils can unwind every tightly coiled nerve. Inhale deeply and the fragrance will fill your psyche with restorative pleasure; touch the key points relating to nerve centers (outlined in Chapters III and IV) and waves of relaxation will course through your entire nervous system. Particularly relaxing essences are lavender, vetiver, ylang-ylang, chamomile, marjoram, basil, and neroli. (See Appendix I for precise formulas.)

### Allergies

An allergy is an unbalanced reaction to the environment, and to substances we either eat, contact via the air, or apply to the skin. An allergy can be a case of overload. You can become allergic to even a healthful substance if you eat it too often. Eating the same food day after day—even an innocuous food, like apricots or potatoes—can so saturate your cells with that substance that they will no longer tolerate any more of it. Try to vary your diet so that you don't eat the same food every day. Supplements that build up your immune system, like pantothenic acid (a B vitamin) and vitamin C, are also helpful. The thymus and adrenal glands are involved in the functioning of the immune system. Pressing these reflex points on the hands and feet can ward off allergies and, if you are allergic, help you to be less so.

The endocrine glands are the body's chief balancers. They control your metabolic rate (the thyroid), your immune system (thymus and adrenals), your blood sugar (pancreas), and hormone production. Working together, the endocrine glands integrate the internal environment and orchestrate the complex functions of every cell in your body and brain. Nurture them with touch, pure essential oils, and a healthful diet and you will live a long, youthful, disease-free life.

### AROMATHERAPY BODY STIMULATING

Every cell in your body—all 75 to 100 trillion of them—is a small world unto itself. Each contains vital components—like chromosomes, genes, DNA, organelles, mitochondria, enzymes, hormones, amino acids, and many other known and unknown elements—that create and maintain life. Every cell can be thought of as a minute power station with an energy supply that works for or against you, depending on the fuel this station is fed.

Circulation, the movement of the blood, lymph, and oxygen through the body and brain, is an important key to cell stimulation. When circulation is running at its peak, your cells are oxygen-rich and happy. These individual power stations of energy and information build, ingest, digest, eliminate, and otherwise run you more efficiently than your conscious intelligence ever could. However, when what is circulating contains toxic material—such as ammonia compounds, caused by eating too much meat, and letting it sit in the colon—the cells can be irritated and begin to malfunction in numerous ways, including becoming cancerous.

To keep your cells properly stimulated, then, you will first want to clean up what is going to reach them through the circulation process, then work on the circulatory system itself. You can do that by following my Aromatherapy body cleansing suggestions discussed at the beginning of this chapter, and then by adding movement, breathing exercises, and massage to your life.

### Movement

I was a dancer on television and the stage in my teens and twenties, and I had many years of study with the finest instructors in movement, dance, yoga, and calisthenics. My early training taught me the importance of exercise and helped me to keep it a pleasurable and important part of my life. You should select an exercise system and practice it regularly. I begin every day with two hours of walking, yoga, and ballet barre exercises, which set me up for the next fifteen hours of intense activity. I feel more tired, not less, at the end of a day if I don't work out in the morning, and much more tense. Physical exercise is a great relaxer, as well as stimulator, and relaxation is also essential to good circulation. Tension is a powerful vein constrictor, which is why perpetually tense people are heart attack prone. When the arteries close and blood can't get through to the heart or brain, you have the perfect environment for a heart attack or stroke.

Aromatherapists recommend pursuing exercise in a natural way, working to your limits, without pushing beyond your capacity. June Seymour, a movement therapist who works with the Arcier salon in London, advises her exercise students, "Protect your back." It is important to protect your back during all kinds of exercise, as nothing causes more agony and pain than a crippling back injury. Unfortunately, some of the popular forms of exercise today do not make it easy to practice back protection. Jogging and aerobic dance, for example, can damage the back and legs, and jolt the female organs. Too many joggers have dropped organs and chronic shin splints from pounding down on hard-surfaced roads. And too few aerobic dance instructors teach their students about proper body alignment or give sufficient warm-up exercises. Fast walking is one of the best, most natural forms of all-over body exercise, especially if you breathe deeply and consciously.

### Breathing

Breathing is a process that supports every human function, and is therefore an important part of the Aromatherapy system. Breathing stimulates oxygen consumption and utilization, without which you're dead. You can feed a cell every other nutrient, but if oxygen isn't present a molecule called ATP (adenosine triphosphate) cannot release its vital energy, and you'll have none.

Inhaling brings in fresh, oxygenated air, and exhaling sends out bodily waste in the form of carbon dioxide and other gases. Inhaling feeds and exhaling cleans. The way to make the most of both these actions is to breathe diaphragmatically, or from the diaphragm. The diaphragm is a flat muscle that supports the base of the lungs and presses down, opening up the chest area to let it take in air as you inhale. During the exhalation process, the diaphragm puffs up into a dome shape. When you breathe high in your chest the diaphragm is not fully depressed, and you can't bring in as much air. If you breathe too low, down in the stomach, the lungs do not fill fully either. Breathing from the midsection of the torso is the only way to engage the diaphragm fully.

Regular deep breathing not only brings in the oxygen you need to turn on your cells' power supply, it also stabilizes the rhythm of your body and brain. Yogis use rhythmic breathing to enter meditative states, because four thousand years of practice has taught them that the breath can transport the body and mind into a profound state of calm. Breathing, like Aromatherapy, can calm and stimulate simultaneously.

Before you massage yourself or someone else, take just two minutes to practice deep, diaphragmatic breathing. The best position to feel the correct placement of the breath is lying face down (head to one side, if you haven't got a massage table with an opening for the face), arms akimbo next to each side of the head, and legs slightly spread. Take a deep breath, expanding the solar plexus area, where the diaphragm is located. Hold five counts and exhale as fully as possible, contracting the stomach muscles. If you push your diaphragm against the floor or table, you will feel its position and action better. Try this breathing exercise before you go to sleep, and you will drift off faster and dream deeper. When exercising, breathe in as you move up or out, and exhale as you come in or down. This will make movement easier, and will strengthen your diaphragm and lungs, and the ability of the lungs to expand and contract. When walking, make a game of breathing in for as many steps as you can, hold the breath for half that number, and then exhale for as many steps as possible again. This energetic "breath walking" can increase the benefits of every stride. Deep inhalations also put your sense of smell into full play. Try to identify what it is you are smelling and visualize the object at the same time. This exercise will sharpen your sense of smell and increase your enjoyment of scentual experience.

## _____ AROMATHERAPY BODY NOURISHING _____

Nourishing yourself and those you love is a physical as well as emotional process. Aromatherapy massage, bathing with scented oils, and beauty care provide a special system of holistic nourishment, but you need to support scentual nourishment with good nutrition.

Today we are all bombarded with a huge and bewildering (and often useless) variety of "diets," which are based on everything from chic locations to immunity. This diet mania makes it hard to learn what good nutrition really is, and what foods keep you slim and healthy. After many years of studying the work of well-known doctors, chemists, biologists, and nutritionists, I have settled on a few solid, basic rules that work for me and my clients. They are:

- Chew! You have no teeth in your stomach.
- Proper food combining aids digestion and assimilation.
- Whole food nourishes most completely.
- Live food makes for lively, life-loving people.
- Attitude and atmosphere are digestion and assimilation aids.
- Smelling your food will increase your appreciation and enable you to eat less.
- Using herbs, dried and fresh, improves the taste of food and your digestion.

Before I explain the reasons for these rules, keep in mind that every individual is unique. A diet or nutrition program that agrees with someone else may be wrong for you. Even your organs are not shaped or placed exactly like every other person's. During Aromatherapy massage, I am constantly amazed at how different every body is, not to mention every mind. Give any new nutritional program time to work, perhaps a month (unless you have an immediate bad reaction to it), but if you are not feeling better by then, try something else.

### Sink Your Teeth In

Digestion begins in the mouth. If you don't chew solid food you can never digest it completely. Even juices should be held as long as possible in the mouth with a little chewing motion before swallowing. Ideally you should chew every bite you eat until it is liquid. Not only is chewing good for digestion, but saliva is a strong antiseptic that helps to kill harmful bacteria in food. A significant portion of the vitamins and minerals in what you eat are also absorbed in the mouth, and then travel from there into the system. So chew!

### Combine Compatible Foods

The theory of food combining is controversial, and you (and your doctor) may not agree with it. Aromatherapists, as well as nutritionists, however, are now recommending compatible eating as an ideal way to achieve health and weight loss. Eating compatibly means that you do not mix proteins and starches, nor do you mix acids and starches. In other words, the all-American meat and potatoes diet becomes taboo when you practice food combining. Strange though it may sound, this system is based on the exhaustive research of an amazing American doctor, William Howard Hay. Dr. Hay discovered that incomplete digestion loaded the body with toxins, which in turn lowered its defenses against disease. My mother heard of Dr. Hay's work when I was very ill with a mastoid infection at the age of ten. She was told by three doctors that if I wasn't operated on immediately (this was before the era of "miracle" drugs), I would probably contract spinal meningitis and die. My mother ignored this well-meant advice and had the courage to contact Dr. Hay, who she'd read could cure serious infections and arthritis with fasting and compatible eating. Dr. Hay told my mother to give me water and juice until my fever dropped, and then bring me to his Pennsylvania sanitorium. After six weeks with Dr. Hay my ears were clear for the first time in three years. That was the start of my lifelong belief in natural healing. Nothing convinces you like the banishing of excruciating pain.

The principle of the Hay compatible eating system is logical and simple. Starches are almost entirely digested in the mouth by an enzyme called *ptyalin*. Proteins and acids, on the other hand, are digested in the stomach by *hydrochloric acid* and *pepsin*. If you eat proteins and starches together, Dr. Hay has shown, neither is completely digested, and both sit in the stomach, causing digestive problems and creating toxins. Eventually years of incomplete digestion may create other degenerative conditions.

Proteins must have a strong, acid environment; otherwise the pepsin cannot break them down. Starch needs an alkaline medium, which ptyalin in the mouth provides. This is another reason to chew your food well—starch is digested by saliva enzymes. This is also the reason why babies who have not yet teethed can't handle refined carbohydrates, and shouldn't be fed cereals until they can chew. When a starch is eaten with protein, it alkalizes the digestive medium, meaning the protein never gets fully processed.

If you want to test this theory on yourself, make up a list of protein, starch, acid, and neutral foods, or buy a chart that lists them at a health food store. Try the combining system for a month and see if your health improves. You may never need a Tums again. Here is a brief list of food categories.

| PROTEIN | STARCH | ACID | NEUTRAL |
|---|---|---|---|
| Meat | Cereals | Fruits | Green vegetables |
| Fish | Potatoes | Tomatoes | Avocados |
| Eggs | Rice | (*cooked*) | Fats and oils |
| Dairy products | Pasta | Vinegar | Nuts |

Combine proteins with neutral and acid foods, and starches only with neutrals. Once you identify what food falls into what category, the system is easy to follow. Of course, if a Big Mac, solid protein on a starch roll, is your favorite food, you won't love this diet. But your body will—so give it a try. You will also find that food combining automatically eliminates a lot of junk food and fattening treats, and helps you lose weight by asking you to consume less at one sitting.

### Eat the Whole Food

The main reason many of us have to supplement our diet with vitamins and minerals is that these vital elements have been lost in our refined and processed modern food. Dr. Richard Passwater, a recognized authority on vitamin E, traces the current high incidence of heart disease back to the time wheat germ was taken out of flour. Vitamin E, contained in wheat germ and not in breads made from white flour, is intimately involved in bringing oxygen to the cells and keeping the arteries open.

No matter how much our food is "enriched," or how many supplements we take, there is no substitute for eating the food the way nature grows it— whole. Every natural food contains not only its own particular combination of nourishing vitamins, minerals, enzymes, and other chemicals, but also trace elements that enable it to be digested and assimilated, or used by your system. For example, the vitamin C supply in an orange is absorbed much better if the bioflavonoids found in the orange's membranes are eaten with it. If you drink orange juice you miss the bioflavonoids. There's nothing wrong with orange juice (unless it's a commercial brand loaded with sugar), but the whole orange is better.

The health-destroying ingredient consumed everywhere in the world today is white sugar. Everything that chemically balances cane sugar is removed in the refining process, which is why sugar, and everything with sugar in it, is digested so briefly and causes blood sugar problems.

Even if you go to the effort to find and eat healthy whole grains, natural sugars, and unprocessed fruits, vegetables, animal proteins, and dairy products, it's still wise to take a wide-spectrum vitamin/mineral supplement. This is necessary because the earth our food is nourished on is no longer whole. Fertilizers and pesticides have changed the structure of the soil itself to the point where some absolutely vital minerals, like selenium, are completely eliminated. If they're not in the soil, they're usually not in the food; so eat whole food, and then make it even more whole with a good supplement.

### Eat Living Food

Just as I believe in the natural life force of pure essential oils, I believe in the power of food that contains live enzymes. Live food means raw food. Though I won't suggest that you eat all your food raw (some things, like grains, are better for you cooked), I definitely advise not cooking everything you eat.

Raw foods and juices have been used since Hippocrates for healing as well as for building health. One of the world's most respected and successful nutritionists, Swiss physician Max Bircher-Benner, created a system in the late 1800s of restoring health based on raw foods and vegetable juices. People still flock to his clinic from many countries. Cooking not only destroys valuable enzymes that aid digestion and assimilation, it also does away with many vitamins, especially water-soluble B and C. Some important amino acids are also destroyed in cooking protein. Heating unsaturated fats to a high temperature can be dangerous, as well, because high heat changes the molecular structure of unsaturates, creating "free radicals." These free radicals can cause cell changes, a precursor to cancer. It's better to cook with butter or olive oil (which is both a saturate and unsaturate), than with safflower and sunflower oils.

One of the most effective and pleasant ways to meet your raw quotient is with freshly extracted vegetable juices. Raw carrots are hard to chew and digest because they're so fibrous, but you can drink three carrots in a moment, and send all that nourishing vitamin A into the digestive tract quickly. Juice extractors are now reasonably priced and available in all department and health food stores. There are a good many books on making juices, including those by Dr. Norman Walker, a gentleman I had the honor to meet when he was in his prime at 77. Dr. Walker lived to be 114, and when he died he was still writing, gardening, and studying Sanskrit—a living testimony to the power of raw vegetable juices, which he consumed at every meal.

If you have been existing (and I use the word advisedly) mostly on cooked food, don't instantly convert to mostly raw food. The fibers and enzymes in the living food will stir up large amounts of residue in the colon, and you will be headachy as well as gassy. Just add an extra raw salad and a glass of vegetable juice to your daily fare for a while. Eventually, you can get to the point where 50 percent (or even better, 75 percent) of your diet is composed of life-giving raw foods.

### Eat in a Nourishing Atmosphere
Your state of mind when you eat is almost as important as what you eat. Tension has a negative effect on digestive juices and inhibits their flow. You should try to be as calm and positive as possible to get the most out of every morsel. Setting an attractive table actually helps your food help you. If you are alone, spoil yourself by dining by candlelight with soft music playing. Aren't you worth it? Don't eat something you hate simply because you think it's good for you; it probably won't do you much good at all since negative emotions will block its absorption. I studied nutrition with Paavo Airola, author of seventeen books on health and nutrition; he told me that all over the world people celebrated holidays by breaking their usual dietary routines and eating and drinking different food, and more of it, for a day or so. He advised his students, who strictly followed his vegetarian regime, to kick over the traces once a month and eat forbidden fare. The result, as I discovered, is that you usually don't feel very well after your celebration, and it makes you really appreciate your normal routine. Airola also theorized that sending your body some radically different food would wake up your

immune system while adding some unexpected fun to your life. Whatever you eat, it's important to remember that food should be fun as well as nourishing.

### Delight in the Aroma of Food

Our sense of taste and our sense of smell are so intimately related that when one malfunctions so does the other. Smell and taste also enhance one another. Consciously smelling your food will add an extra dimension of enjoyment to the eating process, and stimulate your digestive juices. Savor the fragrance of food before you start to eat; the enticing aromas will activate your salivary glands. You may also find that since you are giving more than just one sense the dining experience, you will be satisfied with less food. You can savor your calories with your nose, and never gain an ounce.

### Cook with Aromats

Since ancient man began to cook, aromats, or fragrant herbs and spices, have been used to flavor and to preserve. The modern cook is fortunate to have a wide range of fresh aromatic herbs and spices available in every supermarket. With only a teaspoon of dried, or two teaspoons of fresh, herbs, you can transform a pedestrian dish into a gourmet treat. The addition of aromats also aids digestion, as spices and herbs titillate the sense of taste and smell.

Vinegars are vastly improved by adding dried or fresh dill, tarragon, basil, or rosemary. When adding dried herbs, heat the vinegar to near boiling. Fresh herbs should be macerated or pounded, and let sit for a while in lukewarm vinegar. Sage helps remove the acidity of tomatoes. Rosemary, used in soup or rubbed into lamb, will purify the food as well as your digestive tract. Marjoram changes the flavor of mushrooms, making them sweeter and more flavorful, and has a calming effect on your digestion. Garlic is not only a powerful seasoning, it contains alicin, a natural antibiotic, which parasites and bacteria hate.

Today, most health-oriented people are cutting down the fat and salt in their diets; aromatics can take their place in a beneficial and delicious way. Experiment with fresh herbs, such as parsley, chives, and dill, in salads and omelettes instead of salt. Sauté vegetables in a little water with a touch of dried basil or rosemary, instead of butter. Fish is marvelous if marinated for two hours in sage, rosemary, thyme, and lemon juice, then quickly broiled. Large fresh basil leaves, both cooked and raw, add decorative flavor and fragrance to dishes; try them on big tomato slices. Fresh or dried, aromats make you a scentual cook.

## ____ THE AROMATHERAPY DIET _____

From the Aromatherapy viewpoint, a body that is functioning in balance is seldom over- or underweight. The desire for too much food and no desire for food at all are not normal, human conditions. If you are too fat or too thin, Aromatherapy, with its body balancing and toning techniques, can help you to achieve and maintain a normal weight. The massage relaxes and decongests the body, while the essential oils tone the skin and uplift the mood. (Depression can too often lead to overweight, and vice versa.)

There are three major causes of overweight: (1) water retention due to excess salt in the diet or perhaps an inherited inability to eliminate fluid; (2) increase in fat tissue due to excessive eating; and (3) biological water retention due to nervous tension or shock (stress can block the lymph thereby hindering the elimination of toxic fluids and water). In all cases the basic massage and self-massage as well as the bathing suggestions in Chapters III, IV, and VI can put you on the road to scentual slimness. If too much water or fat is covering the tissues, work on key pressure points that stimulate the glands on the hands, feet, and head. Below are additional recommendations that should alleviate each overweight condition:

### 1. Water Retention
*Oils to use in massage and bath*: Geranium, cypress, and juniper
*Teas*: Uva ursi (very diuretic), comfrey, dandelion, and alfalfa
*Eliminate from diet*: Salt and salty foods, fats, and refined carbohydrates
*Include in diet*: Vitamin/mineral supplement with 500 milligrams of extra C (C is a diuretic)

### 2. Increase in Fat Tissue

*Oils to use in massage and bath*: Lavender, rosemary, thyme, sage, and sandalwood

*Teas*: Peppermint, lemongrass, and sage

*Eliminate from diet*: Fats, salt, refined carbohydrates and sugars, alcohol, processed food, and very high caloric food such as nuts, avocado, and fatty meats

*Include in diet*: Vitamin/mineral supplement plus kelp tablets if blood pressure is not high and you do not have acne (iodine seems to promote acne), vegetables and their juices (as many raw as possible), complex carbohydrates with no butter, lean fish and meat, boiled or poached eggs (not fried or scrambled), and small amount of fresh fruit, except bananas

### 3. Tense Tissue Weight

*Oils to use in massage and bath*: Lavender, chamomile, basil, vetiver, and neroli

*Teas*: Chamomile, rosehip, verbena, and lime blossom

*Eliminate from diet*: Fats, salt, refined carbohydrates and sugars, alcohol, and processed food

*Include in diet*: Vitamin/mineral supplement with added B and pantothenic acid (perhaps 100 milligrams of each B vitamin), brewer's yeast and wheat germ, vegetables and their juices (as many raw as possible), complex carbohydrates, nonfat dairy products, lean fish and meat, boiled or poached eggs, small amount of fresh fruit, including bananas, some raw, fresh nuts for the magnesium

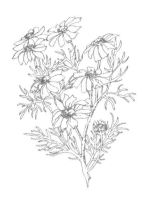

# AROMATHERAPY FOR PREGNANCY AND BABY CARE

Pregnancy can be both an emotionally fulfilling and a demanding condition. On one hand you contemplate the miracle of bringing a new life into this world; on the other, your body and emotions are careening through changes that can make you achy, nauseous, fatigued, nervous, and slightly crazy.

Here are some touch techniques that can relieve tension and discomfort. They can be done by a loving husband or a supportive friend.

Since pregnant women are usually uncomfortable lying on their stomachs after the first three months, a seated position works better for massage of the neck and back, two areas that become especially tired and tense during pregnancy. Ask the pregnant woman to sit on the edge of a table with her feet up on a stool. If it's chilly, surround her with a blanket, leaving only the area to be worked on bare. A pillow placed on the knees in front of her abdomen will give comfort and support when you are working on the back.

### Polarity Presses
The body-balancing polarity holds are particularly beneficial for pregnant women, since they can stimulate and calm without even touching the body. Use as many holds as the pregnant woman finds comfortable. These are outlined in Chapter V.

### Relieving the Base of the Head
Stand in front of the pregnant woman, holding her head in your hand. (See Illustration IX–1.) With the other hand, trace a line across the base of the skull, massaging in little circles from one side to the other. Repeat six times.

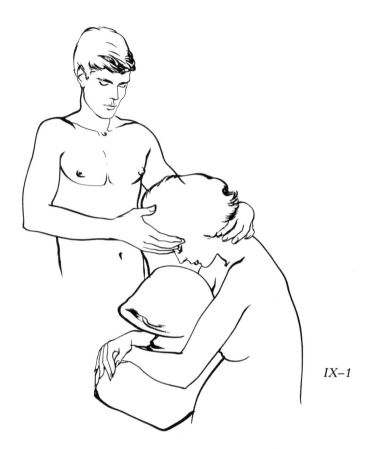

IX–1

*Releasing the Shoulder and Neck*
The additional weight of enlarged breasts results in neck and shoulder tension for many pregnant women. Stand in back of her, and massage the tense area deeply with your fingers. (See Illustration IX–2.)

*Decongesting the Spinal Nerves*
Stand behind the pregnant woman and work up and down the back on each side of the spinal column with your thumbs. Travel up and down five times in each direction. (See Illustration IX–3.) This will relieve the nerves that communicate to the organs, as well as relax the back. After the thumb movements, sweep up the back with the entire surface of both hands with

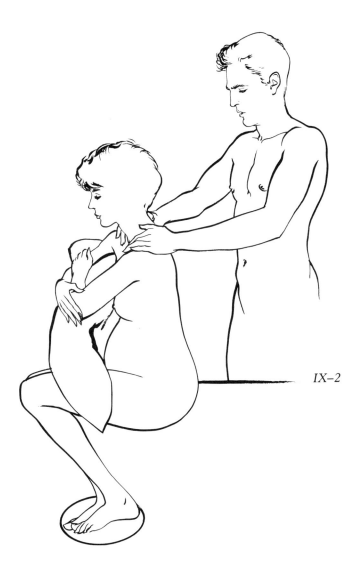

*IX–2*

a soothing effleurage stroke.

## ESSENTIAL OILS FOR PREGNANCY MASSAGE

A few drops of a mild essential oil adds to the uplifting experience of massage, especially needed when pregnant spirits are flagging. Use a rich carrier oil mixture, such as 2 ounces of sesame or soy oil with 1 ounce each of avocado

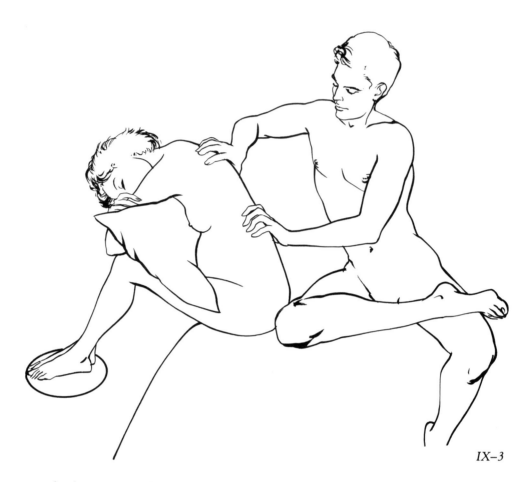

IX–3

and wheat germ oil; this rich carrier oil can be very useful for stretched skin on the pregnant woman's abdomen and breasts. Then add *half* the amount of essence normally recommended; this will generally give you 6 drops in 4 ounces of oil. Because the pregnant system is so volatile, and another life is gestating within it, it is best to be cautious about anything a pregnant woman takes inside or applies to her body. Gentle floral essences like lavender, rose, geranium, and chamomile are best. Tangerine oil is also excellent since it treats the skin with vitamin C. The pregnant woman should *not* be massaged with the stronger herbals, like rosemary, thyme, sage, bay, or basil. A mild herb tea, like rosehip, chamomile, or peppermint, is helpful for fatigue and nausea. Peppermint relieves morning sickness.

## ___ THE SCENTUAL BABY _____

Babies need to be touched with love and sensitivity as much as they need other forms of nourishment. Aromatherapy touches, which can help to balance the baby's developing system and encourage optimum growth, should be done with a light but firm hand and a special aromatic baby oil, which you can make yourself.

### BABY MASSAGE OIL

Most commercial baby oils are made with mineral oil, which can eventually prove drying to a baby's skin. You can make a lovely, natural baby oil that will keep your baby from chafing and developing diaper rash and other skin problems by combining sweet almond oil (available in health food stores and bath supply stores) with rose or chamomile. This should be a weak essential-oil mix, so add only 2 drops of essence to 6 ounces of oil. Baby skin is very delicate.

### BABY MASSAGE

#### Calming Sweep

Put the baby on its stomach. With the right hand hold its buttocks and with the left slowly sweep down the middle of the back. (See Illustration IX–4.) Repeat five times.

#### Tummy Rock

Turn the baby over on its back. Hold the left hand on its chest and with the right hand flat on the stomach *gently* rock the baby from side to side. (See Illustration IX–5.) This is more of a jiggle than a rock and should only be done for about thirty seconds. If the baby seems delighted, which most are by this move, repeat several times.

#### Extremity Extensions

With the baby still on its back, take the arms and fold them across the chest, then pull out until they are fully extended and fold in again. Most babies

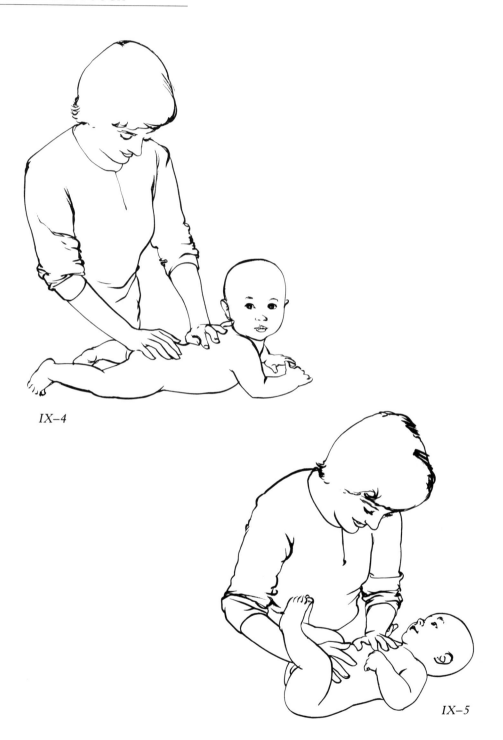

IX–4

IX–5

will think this is a funny game and will giggle. Do the whole movement about five times. The same motion is good for the legs. Hold the ankles and bend the legs into the stomach, then pull them straight out. Repeat five times. This move gives the baby's developing limbs a good stretch and allows any cramped muscles to relax. This, like all the baby moves, should be done gently, with sensitivity and loving eye contact.

### Foot Massage

As tiny as a baby's feet are, they still hold the body contact points illustrated on the foot chart in Chapter IV. You can stimulate the baby's entire system by stroking and touching the feet. (See Illustration IX–6.) Running your thumbs up the top of the foot as described in the basic massage in Chapter IV will wake up the baby's system, making the baby happy and calm.

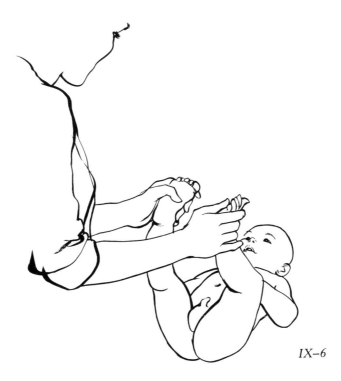

IX–6

### AROMA BABY BATH

Your baby should take naturally to water, since it just emerged from a nine-month swim. When you bathe the baby, let it float a bit, balanced on your hand, which is stretched under its head and shoulders. This post-partum float will be even better for the baby's skin if you add a cup of chamomile tea to the water.

### THE SCENTUAL NURSERY

The purifying fragrance of essential oils can improve the nursery atmosphere while introducing the infant to pleasurable natural aromas. Oil can be dispensed by heat, as suggested in Chapter III, or put a small ball of cotton saturated in essence out of the baby's reach, perhaps behind the padding of the crib. Good oils to use both for purifying and for the baby's delight are lavender, incense, and neroli. If the baby has a cold or cough, pine will help eliminate germs and keep nasal passages open.

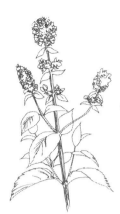

*APPENDIX I*

# SCENTUAL RECIPES

As you mix and match essential oils, you will develop a nose for aromatic compatibility. Though two particular essences may each have a positive effect, they do not necessarily mesh well together. You can tell by the odor when a mixture doesn't match—either it smells "wrong" or one essence knocks out the other, and the mixture loses its distinctive aroma. A mixture combining a floral geranium, a citrus tangerine, and a light herb like sage would smell compatible, whereas a strong, heavy vetiver, a sharp rosemary, and a light, citrusy neroli would be out of balance, because the first two essences would fight for dominance and smother the last. The recipes in this recipe section, as well as those throughout the book, should help you educate your essence sense.

## STORING AND HANDLING ESSENTIAL OILS

Essential oils are expensive and perishable; they require tender loving care. Store them away from light and heat, preferably in dark glass containers. Light will eventually break down these volatile aromatics, and plastic interacts with their chemistry. A high concentration of essences in any mixture of oils will pull plastic into the formula, and collapse the bottle as well as destroy the oil. The bottle cap, however, can be lined with a special kind of plastic that is used for its stability.

Always remember to keep your bottles tightly closed when you aren't using them. Oils are quickly affected by air, and their potency will be significantly reduced if exposed for long. Never leave the bottle cap off longer than it takes to pour the oil into your hand or mix your formulas. Also be sure that the container holding your mixtures is both clean and dry. A single drop of water will cloud essential oils and diminish their performance.

## MIXING THE OILS

Making a mixture requires precise measurements and careful handling of the ingredients. Keep your recipes *simple*. If one or two essences will do the job, there is no point in using six. Home mixing is best done in the kitchen or the bathroom, where spills can be easily mopped up.

Gather all your utensils together before you open the essences; this will minimize exposure of the oils to the air. You will need a measuring cup or beaker, small funnels, and eyedroppers. All should be very clean and dry, and kept covered when not in use. It is best to have a separate dropper and funnel for each essence, so that one essence doesn't pick up the character of the other from the utensils you are using. Try to find tinted bottles in 1- and 4-ounce sizes. The 1-ounce size is good for the pure essences and face oil. Use the 4-ounce size for the mixtures you use in body massage. A larger bottle is hard to handle with oily hands, and exposes your essences over time to a lot of destructive air.

## CARRIER OILS

The essences are mixed with excellent-quality vegetable oils called *carriers*, which can be bought where natural foods are sold. The carriers you buy should be unprocessed, cold-pressed oils that have not been chemically treated. These oils are more perishable than supermarket oils, and you must let your nose be your guide to their freshness. They should have a mild smell, without a trace of rancidity. Once they are opened, keep them in the refrigerator, until you add the aromatics. Since essential oils are antibacterial, they act as preservatives for about six months.

My favorite blend for body massage is a mixture of ⅔ soybean oil with

¹/₃ sesame oil. If a richer blend is needed for dry skin or the face, I mix ¹/₃ soy oil with ¹/₃ almond oil and ¹/₃ avocado oil. Sunflower and safflower oils are good mixers, but since they are lighter and not as lubricating, I tend to use them for summer massage. For mature facial skin I add 10 percent wheat germ oil to any mixture. The vitamin E content of this nourishing oil acts as an antioxidant, and helps preserve both the carrier oils and the essences.

### *The Ratios*

The ratio of essential to carrier oil for the body should be 6 drops of essential oil for every 2 ounces of carrier. I use only 4 drops of essential oil for facial preparations, since the skin on the face is very sensitive. The amount of essential oil you use, however, can vary with individual conditions and needs. Sometimes I have used up to 20 drops of essence per ounce of body oil for a treatment. The requirements and preferences of the person you are massaging will be your guide; but remember, a little essence goes a long way, and even a very good thing can be overdone.

## RECIPES FOR SPECIAL PROBLEMS

Here are remedies using essential oils and herbal teas that can help you cope with life's challenges to health and comfort. To keep things simple as well as effective, I have limited most of the recipes to just two or even one oil at a time. Where the formulas say lavender/chamomile *or* geranium/sandalwood, use either the first or the second combination but not all together, otherwise your mixtures will be too strong. If you find that even these relatively mild doses are in any way irritating to the skin, cut the number of drops in half, or change to an alternative formula. Except for treating a very small area, lavender is the only essence I would use on the skin neat, unless you have had practice with the oils.

### *ACNE*

*Camphor/Lavender*
OR
*Cypress/Lemon*

—These combinations are good for most "spots" as well as acne. In this case use just one drop neat on the lesion.

## ANXIETY/TENSION

*Basil/Neroli*
OR
*Vetiver/Lavender*

⁀ 6 drops each in 4 ounces of carrier oil. Massage in a counterclockwise circle on solar plexus with *left* hand (the calming hand).
⁀ 10 drops each in tub of warm water. Soak for ten minutes.

## ARTHRITIS/RHEUMATISM

*Rosemary/Chamomile*
OR
*Eucalyptus/Sandalwood*

⁀ 6 drops each in 4 ounces of carrier oil. Massage into affected area.
⁀ 10 drops each in tub of warm water. Soak for ten minutes.

## BRONCHITIS, COLDS, FLU

*Pine/Eucalyptus*
OR
*Camphor/Sandalwood*

⁀ 10 drops in 4 ounces of carrier oil. Massage on chest.
⁀ 20 drops each in tub of hot water. Soak ten minutes.
⁀ 15 drops each in 1 quart of hot water. Put towel over head, close eyes, and inhale as long as is comfortable.

## BURNS (Minor)

*Lavender*
OR
*Lavender/Aloe Vera Gel*

⁀ Serious burns should be treated by a physician. However, for minor burns use a drop of lavender neat on burn or mix 4 drops of lavender with 1 teaspoon of aloe vera gel and spread on affected area.

## CELLULITE

*Cypress/Juniper*

⁀ 10 drops each in 4 ounces of carrier oil. Massage well into affected area.
⁀ 20 drops each in warm bath, soak for ten minutes.

## CONSTIPATION

*Rosemary/Thyme*
OR
*Marjoram/Juniper*

⁀ 6 drops each in 4 ounces of carrier oil. Massage counterclockwise on solar plexus. Massage stomach area, up the right side, across the top and down the left in a circular motion to stimulate peristalsis.

## DEPRESSION

*Basil/Neroli*
OR
*Marjoram/Ylang-Ylang*

⁀ 6 drops each in 4 ounces of carrier oil. Massage counterclockwise on solar plexus with left hand.
⁀ 20 drops each in tub of warm water. Soak for ten minutes.

## FATIGUE/EXHAUSTION

*Juniper/Lavender*
OR
*Rosemary/Geranium*

〜 6 drops each in 2 ounces of carrier oil. Massage solar plexus in a counterclockwise circular motion with *right* hand (the stimulating hand).
〜 20 drops each in tub of warm water, soak for ten minutes.
〜 10 drops each in 2 quarts of warm water for foot soak. Soak for ten minutes. Good when you haven't time for a full bath.

## FEVER

*Eucalyptus/Lavender*
OR
*Peppermint*

〜 6 drops each of eucalyptus and lavender or 12 drops of peppermint in 4 ounces of carrier oil. Massage counterclockwise on solar plexus and upper back (preferably simultaneously with your hands corresponding front to back).
〜 10 drops each of eucalyptus and lavender or 20 of peppermint in 1 quart of cool water. Mix well and soak small towel in mixture. Hold on forehead, soak again, then hold on chest. Repeat several times on each area.

## GOUT

*Juniper/Rosemary*

〜 6 drops each in 4 ounces of carrier oil. Apply to affected area and massage counterclockwise on solar plexus.
〜 10 drops each in 2 quarts of cool water for gouty foot soak.

## HAIR LOSS

*Bay/Lavender*
OR
*Sage/Thyme*

〜 6 drops each in 4 ounces of warm carrier oil. Massage into scalp. Absorb for twenty minutes. Shampoo with 3 drops of bay in shampoo.

## HEADACHE

*Peppermint*
OR
*Chamomile*
OR
*Lavender*
OR
*Rosemary*

〜 12 drops of one oil in 4 ounces of carrier oil. Massage around temples, base of skull, and counterclockwise on solar plexus with left hand.
〜 20 drops of one oil in 1 quart of hot water. Put towel over head and inhale as long as is comfortable.

## HEMORRHOIDS

Cypress/Chamomile
OR
Lavender/Juniper

⌐ 20 drops each in tub of hot water. Mix well into water with hand. This should be a shallow sitz soak. Sit for ten minutes.

⌐ 2 drops of lavender and 1 drop of geranium in 1 ounce of carrier oil. Apply to hemorrhoid after soak and after each stool.

## IMPOTENCE

Patchouli/Sandalwood
OR
Clary Sage/Ylang-Ylang

⌐ 6 drops each in 4 ounces of carrier oil. Massage counter-clockwise on solar plexus with right hand.

⌐ Burn as room fragrance next to bed.

## INDIGESTION/GAS

Basil/Chamomile
OR
Peppermint

⌐ 6 drops each basil and chamomile or 12 of peppermint in 4 ounces of carrier oil. Massage on stomach and counter-clockwise with left hand on solar plexus.

⌐ Drink peppermint, chamomile, fennel, or comfrey tea on empty stomach.

## INFECTIONS (Small Cuts and Wounds)

Lavender/Thyme/
Eucalyptus

⌐ 3 drops each in 1 tablespoon of edible quality oil, such as almond. Pat on wound. Lavender can be dropped neat directly on wound.

## INSECT BITES AND STINGS

Lavender/Thyme
OR
Basil/Marjoram
OR
Clay
OR
Neat Lavender

⌐ 3 drops each in 2 tablespoons of carrier oil. Apply to area affected. Lavender can be dropped neat on the area, or smooth a pure clay paste on the bite and leave on until the application wears off by itself.

## INSECT REPELLENT

Lemon/Clove
OR
Geranium/Eucalyptus
OR
Peppermint

⌐ 10 drops each in 4 ounces of carrier oil. Pat on areas likely to be bitten.

⌐ Burn these oils neat in areas where insects congregate.

## KIDNEYS/URINARY INFECTIONS

*Eucalyptus/Sandalwood*
OR
*Juniper/Thyme*

⌐6 drops each in 4 ounces of carrier oil. Massage counter-clockwise on solar plexus with right hand and on mid-back kidney points.
⌐20 drops each in tub of hot water. Soak for ten minutes. A shallow sitz bath is also useful.

## MENOPAUSE

*Chamomile/Sage*
OR
*Cypress/Lavender*

⌐6 drops each in 4 ounces of carrier oil massaged counter-clockwise on solar plexus with right hand.
⌐20 drops each in tub of warm water. Soak for ten minutes.
⌐Drink sage and chamomile tea or uva ursi if retaining water. Make sure nutrition and vitamin/mineral program is good, especially $B_6$, C, E, calcium, and magnesium.

## MENSTRUAL CRAMPS

*Cypress/Sage*
OR
*Chamomile/Marjoram*

⌐6 drops each in 4 ounces of carrier oil massaged counterclockwise on solar plexus with left hand. Gently massage lower stomach over ovaries, and lower back in corresponding area.
⌐Drink chamomile and sage tea.

## MIGRAINE

*Lavender/Eucalyptus*
OR
*Rosemary/Chamomile*
OR
*Peppermint*

⌐6 drops each in 4 ounces of carrier oil. Massage at temples and press headache points illustrated on page 152. Massage solar plexus, and hand and foot points illustrated on page 95 and page 93.
⌐20 drops each in warm bath. Soak for ten minutes.

## NERVOUS SYSTEM (*Balancing*)

*Cypress/Lavender*
OR
*Rosemary/Sage*

⌐6 drops each in 4 ounces of carrier oil. Massage solar plexus counterclockwise with right hand.
⌐Run thumbs up the sides of spine as far as you can go. Press across base of skull six times on each side. Work on foot nerve points illustrated on page 93.
⌐20 drops each in tub of warm water. Soak ten minutes.
⌐Drink chamomile and linden tea.

## SINUS

Eucalyptus/Pine
OR
Cypress/Niaouli

⌐ 20 drops each in 2 quarts of hot water. Put towel over head and inhale as long as comfortable.
⌐ Dip the towel in essenced water while still hot and use as compress on sinus area above and between eyebrows. Try to eliminate milk and milk products from diet, since they are mucus forming.

## SKIN, CHAPPED, VERY DRY

Lavender/Sandalwood/
Rose

⌐ 6 drops each in 4 ounces of carrier oil consisting of 2 ounces of soy oil, 1 ounce of almond oil, 1 ounce of avocado oil, and 1 tablespoon of wheat germ oil.

## SUNBURN

Lavender/Chamomile

⌐ 20 drops each in tub of cool water. Soak ten minutes.

## VARICOSE VEINS

Cypress/Geranium

⌐ 12 drops each in 4 ounces of carrier oil. Stroke upward toward heart on affected area. *Do not* massage on the veins, but around them and very gently slide over veins just to apply oil.

Let scentual touch activate your belief system: belief in yourself and the power of nature to light your way.

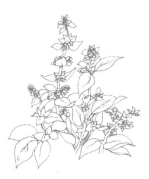

# RESOURCES FOR HERBS AND ESSENCES

Pure essential oils are often available at your local health food store. However, if that is not the case in your area, here are a few direct-mail resources:

Aphrodisia
282 Bleecker Street
New York, NY 10012
(212)989-6440

Bach Flower Remedies
463 Rockaway Avenue
Valley Stream, NY 11580
(516)825-2229

Herbal Educational Center
6 Crescent Road
Burlington, VT 05401

Herbcraft
P.O. Box 352 RD4
Scotland Road
Quarryville, PA 17566
(717)786-1131

Kripalu Shop
Box 774
Lenox, MA 01240
(413)637-3280

L&H Vitamins Inc.
38-01 35th Avenue
Long Island City, NY 11101
(718)937-7400

Living Earth Crafts
429 Olive Street
Santa Rosa, CA 95407
(707)545-6644 or (800)358-8292

Walnut Acres
Penns Creek, PA 17862
(717)837-0601

# FURTHER READING

## AROMATHERAPY

*Aromatherapy for Women* by Maggie Tisserand. Published by Thorsons Publishers, Inc., New York, 1985.

*The Art of Aromatherapy* by Robert B. Tisserand. Published by Destiny Publishing, New York, 1977.

*The Practice of Aromatherapy* by Dr. Jean Valnet. Published by C.W. Daniel Company, Ltd., Saffron Walden, Essex, England, 1982.

## MASSAGE

*Body Reflexology* by Mildred Carter. Published by Parker Publishing Company, Inc., West Nyack, New York, 1983.

*The Book of Dō-In* by Michio Kushi. Published by Japan Publications, Elmsford, New York, 1979.

*Do-It-Yourself Shiatsu* by Wataru Ohashi. Published by E.P. Dutton, New York, 1976.

*Hand Reflexology* by Mildred Carter. Published by Parker Publishing Company, Inc., West Nyack, New York, 1975.

*Helping Yourself with Foot Reflexology* by Mildred Carter. Published by Parker Publishing Company, Inc., West Nyack, New York, 1969.

*The Joy of Touch* by Dr. Russ A. Rueger. Published by Simon and Schuster, New York, 1981.

*Loving Hands: The Traditional Indian Art of Baby Massage* by Frederick Leboyer. Published by Alfred Knopf, New York, 1982.

*Your Healing Hands: The Polarity Experience* by Richard Gordon. Published by Wingbow Press, Berkeley, California, 1978.

## HEALTH AND BEAUTY

*The Anatomy Coloring Book* by Wynn Kapit/Lawrence M. Elson. Published by Harper and Row, New York, 1977.

*Diet and Nutrition* by Rudolf Ballentine, M.D. Published by The Himalayan Institute, Honesdale, Pennsylvania, 1978.

*Every Woman's Book: Dr. Airola's Practical Guide to Holistic Health* by Paavo Airola, N.D., Ph.D. Published by Health Plus Publishers, Phoenix, Arizona, 1979.

*Fragrance: The Story of Perfume from Cleopatra to Chanel* by Edwin T. Morris. Published by Charles Scribner's Sons, New York, 1984.

*Fit for Life* by Harvey and Marilyn Diamond. Published by Warner Books, New York, 1985.

*Jean Rose's Herbal Body Book* by Jean Rose. Published by Grosset and Dunlap, New York, 1976.

*Food Combining for Health* by Doris Grant and Jean Joyce. Published by Thorsons Publishing Group, New York, 1984.

*Raw Energy* by Leslie and Susannah Kenton. Published by Century Publishing, London, England, 1984.

*The Joy of Beauty* by Leslie Kenton. Published by Doubleday, Garden City, New York, 1983.

*Raw Vegetable Juices* by N.W. Walker, D.Sci. Published by The Berkeley Publishing Group, New York, 1983.

*The Science of Breath* by Swami Rama, Rudolph Ballentine, M.D., Alan Hymes, M.D. Published by The Himalayan Institute, Honesdale, Pennsylvania, 1981.

## MASSAGE TAPE

*Kripalu Meditative Massage.* Prepared by Kripalu Center for Holistic Health, Lenox, Massachusetts.

# *INDEX*